Your Personal Guide

ANGIOPLASTY

Your
Personal Guide

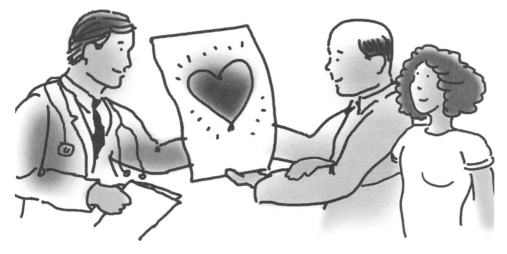

ANGIOPLASTY

Straightforward Answers to Common Questions Every Patient Asks

ALLEN JEREMIAS, MD
and SUSAN S. BARTELL, PsyD

Published by
MPP Publishing, Inc.
666 Old Coutry Road, Suite 602
Garden City, NY 11530

ISBN: 978-0-9857982-0-8

First Printing

Cover design by George Foster
Interior design by Desktop Miracles, Inc.
Illustrations by Megan Rojas
Publisher's Cataloging-In-Publication Data
(Prepared by The Donohue Group, Inc.)
Jeremias, Allen.

   Your personal guide : angioplasty : straightforward answers to common questions every patient asks / Allen Jeremias and Susan S. Bartell.

      p. : ill. ; cm.

   Includes bibliographical references and index.
   ISBN: 978-0-9857982-0-8

   1. Angioplasty—Popular works.   2. Heart—Surgery—Popular works.   3. Heart—Diseases—Popular works.   4. Blood-vessels—Surgery—Popular works.   5. Patient education.   I. Bartell, Susan S. II. Title.   III. Title: Angioplasty
RD598.5 .J47   2012

                                                                    617.412

Printed in the United States of America

Contents

Introduction   1

CHAPTER ONE: **Is This Really Happening to Me?**   3

Question 1   *How do I know it's a heart attack and not something else?*
             What should I do if I think I'm having a heart attack?   4

Question 2   *What actually happened in my body*
             when I had a heart attack?   7

Question 3   *I get chest pain when I exercise, does this mean*
             I'm having a heart attack?   13

Question 4   *I think I'm feeling better. Can I wait a little while*
             before seeing my doctor?   16

Question 5   *How did I get this?*   21

CHAPTER TWO: **The Next Steps: Learning More About My Heart**   27

Question 6   *My family doctor gave me a list of cardiologists.*
             How do I know which one is the best one for me?   28

Question 7   *My cardiologist just told me to get a stress test.*
             What does that mean?   32

Question 8   *I can't walk on a treadmill.*
             Can I still take a stress test?   38

Question 9   *What other tests could my doctor prescribe?*   42

Question 10   *My doctor just gave me my test results.*
              I probably have heart disease. What should I do now?   48

Question 11   *My husband and kids ask me questions about what's going*
              on with my heart, but I don't always remember
              what the doctors told me. How do I get better at that?   54

CHAPTER THREE: **I Just Found Out That I Have Heart Disease** 61

Question 12 *My doctor started me on several medications.*
Will this be enough to cure me? 62

Question 13 *What is a coronary angiogram?* 67

Question 14 *I don't want to admit it, but I'm nervous*
about getting an angiogram. What does it feel like? 74

Question 15 *Now that the procedure is over and I'm recovering,*
are there any precautions I should take? 80

Question 16 *My angiogram showed that I have a blockage in*
my heart artery. What are my options now? 86

CHAPTER FOUR: **Which Treatment Is Right for Me?** 93

Question 17 *Is medication alone enough to make me feel better?* 94

Question 18 *How does a coronary angioplasty work?* 100

Question 19 *How will I feel during this procedure?* 106

Question 20 *My doctor placed a stent in my coronary artery.*
What exactly is a stent? 111

Question 21 *My doctor said I was given a drug-coated stent.*
Is that better? 116

Question 22 *Can anything go wrong during the angioplasty procedure?* 119

Question 23 *Does a stent actually help stop a heart attack?* 125

Question 24 *My blockages cannot be fixed with a stent.*
I need bypass surgery. Then he told me what happens next . . . 129

Question 25 *When can I get back to my regular life?* 136

CHAPTER FIVE: **Learning to Live the *Heart♥SMART®* Way** 141

Question 26 *I'm feeling much better. What's next for me?* 142

Question 27 *My doctor has given me five different medications.*
Isn't this too much? 147

Question 28 *My cholesterol is normal.*
Do I really need cholesterol medication? 152

Question 29 *I have diabetes. Does this make things worse?* 158

Question 30 *My blood pressure is high, but I feel fine.*
Can I manage it without medication? 164

CHAPTER SIX: **You Are Worth It!** 171

Question 31 *My life is stressful, but how does this affect my heart and what should I do about it?* 172

Question 32 *Is it okay to be active after my heart procedure?* 180

Question 33 *My doctor told me to eat healthily. How do I do that?* 189

Question 34 *I've been battling my weight for years, and now my life depends on it. How am I supposed to lose weight now?* 199

Question 35 *Do I have to stop drinking alcohol when I start the Heart♥SMART program?* 205

Question 36 *I know smoking can cause cancer, but what does it have to do with my heart?* 211

A Final Word 221

APPENDIX ONE: **CPR Instructions** 223
APPENDIX TWO: **Resources** 227

References 235
Index 239

About the Authors and Contributors 245

Introduction

Welcome! We are so glad you are here, because this is an opportunity for you to learn all the important information you need to know about taking care of your heart and angioplasty. It is quite normal for you to have many questions about heart disease. By the time you have finished reading, we are confident that most of your questions will have been answered.

The following chapters take you through all the stages of coronary artery disease, from diagnosis through treatment, and the steps you should take to ensure yourself a healthy future. As you will see, each chapter contains questions asked by almost every person who has heart disease and undergoes angioplasty. Throughout the book we will follow five people—Brian, Rosa, Michael, Reginald, and Diane—each of whom probably have some of the same questions that you may have.

We will answer their questions in plain English so it really makes sense to them and to you! Each response is divided into two sections: The Bottom Line and The Nitty Gritty. The Bottom Line contains the most basic and important information that you need to know. You should definitely read The Bottom Line answer for every question. The Nitty Gritty provides additional information for those who would like to understand the response in more detail. The Nitty Gritty information is important, but if you are feeling a bit overwhelmed right now (which is understandable), you can choose to read this section later. Don't worry. This is just fine, because you should learn the information at the pace that works for you.

We are very happy to be able to help you through this stressful and confusing time, and we hope that this book makes your experience just a bit more positive.

To your good health!

Dr. Allen Jeremias and *Dr. Susan Bartell*

One

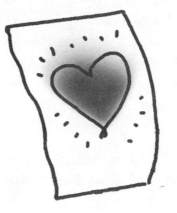

Is This Really Happening to Me?

QUESTION **1** ———————

Brian (53) has high blood pressure and is a smoker. In addition, he has a family history of heart disease. In fact, both his father and his older brother have had heart attacks in their early fifties. However, Brian was still shocked when he had a heart attack.

"I never thought it would happen to me, but two days ago, I suddenly began feeling like I had a ton of bricks weighing on my chest. I struggled to breathe. I started sweating, and my skin felt clammy. I was really scared! As soon as I told my wife, Pat, she panicked and immediately called 911. Thank goodness she did, because the doctor told me that Pat's quick response probably saved my life!

Now that I'm feeling a little better, I can't help wondering . . . "

How do I know it's a heart attack and not something else? What should I do if I think I'm having a heart attack?

THE BOTTOM LINE

Brian was fortunate because he had obvious signs of a heart attack and was able to get help quickly.

The reality is that only about 60 to 70 percent of people have "typical" heart attack symptoms. These include:

- Chest pain or a heavy feeling of pressure on your chest (like the "ton of bricks" Brian described).
- A feeling of severe tightness or squeezing, like a belt being tightened around your chest.
- Shortness of breath with chest pain (Brian felt this too).

- Sweating with or without chest pain (women are less likely than men to experience this, but Brian definitely felt it).
- Clammy skin with or without chest pain (Brian's dad later told him that he had never had the chest discomfort that Brian felt).
- Nausea or vomiting with or without chest pain.
- A feeling that the pain in your chest is radiating from your chest to your neck, jaw, shoulder, or arm (usually your left arm, but not necessarily). Pain in the left arm is the usual way that movies and television show someone to be having a heart attack. However, if you don't feel this, it doesn't mean you are *not* having a heart attack. People have heart attacks with no left-arm pain, and people experience left-arm pain for reasons other than a heart attack. So don't rely on this symptom . . . but don't ignore it either.

You're probably wondering what a heart attack might feel like if you don't experience chest pain or the other typical symptoms. About 30 to 40 percent of people experience atypical symptoms, including

- Chest sensations other than heavy pressure, such as a dull ache or even a sharp pain
- A burning in the chest or upper abdomen that may be mistaken for acid reflux
- Pain in the upper abdomen, neck, jaw, shoulder, or arm without chest pain
- Shortness of breath or heart palpitations without chest pain
- Upper back pain

As you might realize, the symptoms of a heart attack can mimic other—usually less serious—problems, such as heartburn or a panic attack. It can therefore sometimes be difficult to know whether you are actually having a heart attack. In addition, those who have already experienced a heart attack or who have received a stent or other heart procedure are more likely to be sensitive to their body's signals and, understandably, may assume that every symptom is a possible heart attack.

This continual vigilance can be stressful, causing a roller coaster of feelings. Nevertheless, it is important to allow a medical specialist to make the final diagnosis. ***Under all circumstances, it is critical to be cautious and assume that you are having a heart attack, because the quicker you receive treatment, the better your outcome.*** If you are mistaken, the ER doctors and nurses will understand. In fact, they will be happy to tell you the good news that you're not having a heart attack. However, if it is a heart attack, they will be glad you came in early enough to receive treatment that will minimize damage to your heart.

There are four simple rules to follow when you think you or someone else is having a heart attack. These will ensure that you receive help as quickly as possible:

1. Call 911 immediately and wait for the paramedics to arrive. This is the fastest and safest way to get medical attention. Fortunately for Brian, this is exactly what his wife did!
2. *Do not* drive yourself to the emergency room. If you faint while driving, you could seriously injure yourself or others.
3. If you are a bystander, do not drive the person to the ER. If the patient's heart stops, or if he or she stops breathing while you are traveling to the hospital, there is nothing you can do to help. Instead, wait for the ambulance. Emergency responders carry a defibrillator (which can restart a heart). If necessary, the paramedics will use a defibrillator in the ambulance to save the patient's life.
4. If you see that someone else is showing *very* serious signs of a heart attack, including loss of consciousness or severe breathing difficulty, call 911 immediately and then start CPR or chest compressions and continue until help arrives. We have included instructions on how to administer CPR in Appendix 1.

THE NITTY GRITTY

Chest pressure, heaviness, and tightness are actually more specific signs of a heart attack than is actual chest pain. While many things can cause chest pain (including a panic attack), chest pressure, heaviness, and tightness are more often than not caused by a heart attack.

It is well documented that women more frequently experience atypical heart attack symptoms than men (although men may also have them). A recent large study,[1] evaluating nearly 435,000 patients diagnosed with a heart attack, found that up to one-third of these patients did not present with typical chest pain. It is therefore important to learn all the signs of a heart attack that we list here and to try to be in tune with your body's signals.

To make matters just a bit more complicated, it is important to note that up to 15 percent of heart attacks are completely *silent,* which means that they occur with no symptoms or with minimal symptoms that are easy to ignore. Silent heart attacks are more common in people with diabetes, because diabetes affects nerve endings and pain receptors, which may decrease pain sensation. In addition, silent heart attacks are also more common in people over seventy years old, particularly if they have other diseases that may decrease pain sensations or increase tolerance for pain. For example, one may be more likely to experience a silent heart attack when he also has (among other things) Alzheimer's disease or a chronic pain condition.

QUESTION **2**

Rosa (73) was baby-sitting her two grandchildren when she began to feel as if she had acid reflux.

"The kids and I had eaten pizza for lunch, so I assumed this had caused reflux. I also felt nauseous, but I tried to ignore it because I had to take care of my grandbabies. Later that night I noticed a tight feeling in my neck and jaw, and I just couldn't breathe easily. I decided to lie down, thinking I was just tired from running after the kids all day. At about 3 AM, I woke up with crushing chest pain and I couldn't catch my breath at all. I managed to call 911, and then I woke up my husband, Eduardo.

"Thankfully, the ambulance arrived quickly—both Eduardo and I were panicking by then. The EMTs told me that, given my symptoms and the fact that I have diabetes and smoke, I was probably having a heart attack.

"Ever since having this scary experience I've been wondering . . .

What actually happened in my body when I had a heart attack?

THE BOTTOM LINE

A heart attack is caused by a *sudden, complete* blockage (called an occlusion) of one of the blood vessels that supplies blood to the heart muscle. These blood vessels are called coronary arteries (Figure 1), and the term "having a coronary" and the words "heart attack" actually mean the same thing. When a coronary artery is fully occluded, no blood from that artery can reach the heart muscle, and the heart experiences damage.

As you can see from the diagram, coronary arteries are similar to the branches of a tree. The arteries near the trunk are large and become smaller as they move farther away from the trunk. The closer an occlusion is to the "trunk"—or main blood vessel—the greater the potential damage to the heart, because larger arteries cut off a greater

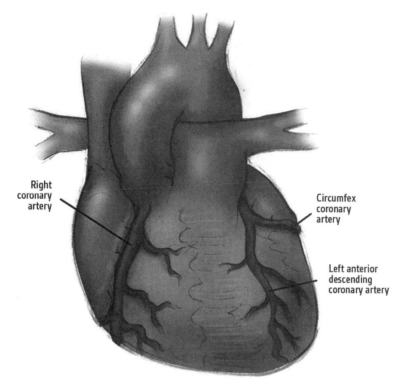

Right
coronary
artery

Circumfex
coronary
artery

Left anterior
descending
coronary artery

Figure 1

supply of blood from the heart. Occlusions in main arteries lead to larger heart attacks and sometimes to sudden death.

What causes an artery to become occluded?

A heart attack usually occurs when an artery is already partially blocked (typically a blockage of less than 70 percent). The partial blockage is caused by a buildup of *plaque* (cholesterol that is deposited into the wall of the blood vessel; see Figure 2). The actual and immediate cause of the heart attack is when a blood clot attaches itself to the partial blockage, causing the artery to become fully occluded. When the blood vessel is fully blocked, the blood flow to the heart muscle is interrupted in the area supplied by the blocked blood vessel. The lack of blood flow to the heart muscle causes the actual heart attack.

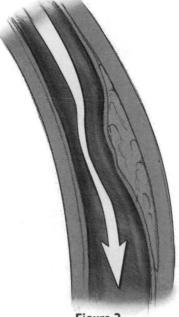

Figure 2

Okay, but why is the "70 percent" important?

In most cases, a blockage of less than 70 percent *will not cause any symptoms,* even when you exercise. In fact, most people eventually have some degree of blockages as they age, and most of these blockages do not cause a heart attack. Under most circumstances, you may not even realize that you have a blocked artery until you are suddenly having a heart attack. On the other hand, when someone has an occlusion of above 70 percent, she is more likely to have warning signs (see Question 3). Seek medical care and avoid a heart attack by taking the right medications or having a procedure (like receiving a stent to open up the partial blockage—more on this later). You might be surprised to learn that about three-quarters of heart attacks begin in vessels with blockages of less than 70 percent, and therefore occur suddenly and without prior warning.

Since heart disease can creep up so quietly, it is best to address risk factors that could lead to heart disease before a heart attack actually occurs.

In Rosa's case, being overweight and not adequately controlling her diabetes or high cholesterol were significant risk factors. In addition, being a woman and having diabetes were two risk factors for her having had atypical symptoms of a heart attack (see Question 1).

It is important for everyone—no matter what the risk—to receive regular medical care and to live a healthy lifestyle (see chapter 6 for some ideas on how to do this). It is also important to pay attention to your body's signals, especially if you have risk factors like Rosa did (overweight, high cholesterol, and diabetic).

Rosa delayed getting medical treatment because she assumed that her symptoms were something less serious. By the time she finally reached the hospital, tests revealed that one coronary artery was completely blocked. Fortunately, the medical team was able to open the vessel with angioplasty and save Rosa's life. Nevertheless, since the blood supply to Rosa's heart muscle had been significantly compromised for some time, Rosa's recovery was slower and not as ideal as it might have been had she sought medical care more quickly. In fact, she suffered considerable damage to her heart muscle because her blockage was not treated quickly enough.

THE NITTY GRITTY

Partial blockages are also called "hardening of the arteries," named for the plaque that is deposited in the artery. Over time, deposits of cholesterol (plaque) cause the inner wall of the artery to thicken, allowing less and less space through which blood can flow. In some people, a large number of white blood cells can infiltrate these plaque deposits. White blood cells typically fight infections and other diseases, but they can also attack cholesterol plaques, leading to "inflammation." You may have experienced inflammation when you have an abscess;

for example, when a cuticle becomes infected. The swelling, redness, and hotness in that area is called inflammation and is caused by an accumulation of white blood cells that fight the infection. When this type of inflammation happens in cholesterol plaque inside a coronary artery, the plaque may become unstable and rupture. The rupture exposes the cholesterol and other plaque particles to the bloodstream, which then leads to the formation of a blood clot right there in the artery. It is this blood clot that leads to the complete occlusion of the artery, causing a heart attack (Figure 3).

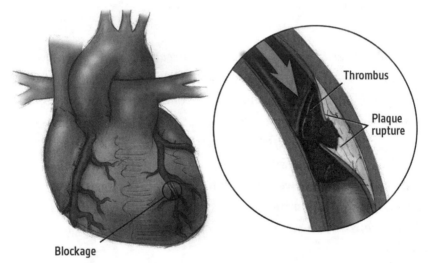

Figure 3

One of the most common questions people ask (sometimes only to themselves!) is, **Can sex cause a heart attack?** The answer: It's rare but it can happen, especially when someone is not in great shape. Interestingly, you face the greatest risk when having sexual relations with a new partner. The psychological excitement of the encounter causes an adrenaline rush, which likely contributes to triggering a heart attack. The moral of this story: if you lead a sedentary lifestyle and you haven't had sexual relations in a while, see your doctor for a heart checkup before engaging in sexual activity.

QUESTION **3** ——————

Michael (64) has always exercised sporadically. Recently he decided to step it up a bit, because his wife and kids have been nagging him to lose a little weight. In addition, at his recent physical exam, the doctor suggested that he lose about thirty pounds in order to control his high blood pressure and elevated cholesterol. When he started to work out on the treadmill, Michael began to feel discomfort in the middle of his chest that felt heavier and heavier as he continued to exercise. At first, he ignored this feeling, but then he noticed that, as he pushed himself to continue, it became more difficult to breathe. As he realized that his symptoms were increasing rather than resolving, Michael became scared. Eventually the pressure in his chest and trouble breathing made it impossible for him to continue. He was relieved to see that about five minutes after getting off the treadmill, the chest pressure was gone and his breathing had improved.

"I really want to exercise and lose some weight, but I'm worried that every time I work out I start to feel bad. It's got me wondering . . . "

I get chest pain when I exercise, does this mean I'm having a heart attack?

THE BOTTOM LINE

In all likelihood, it does *not* mean that you're having a heart attack. While it is possible to have a heart attack during or shortly after exercising (especially if, like Michael, you have just started exercising after being sedentary for a long time), it is more likely that the chest pain or discomfort is caused by a partial blockage in one of your coronary arteries (the blood vessels supplying blood to the heart).

There is a significant difference between a heart attack and a partial blockage. A heart attack is triggered by a complete or almost complete occlusion of an artery, which then causes damage to the area of the heart supplied by that artery—unless the artery is opened immediately (see Question 2).

A partial blockage is typically a 70 to 95 percent blockage (remember from Question 2 that a blockage of less than 70 percent does not usually cause symptoms), allowing for blood flow to continue to the heart muscle.

So if there is still blood flow to my heart, why do I feel pain when I exercise?

Good question! Under most circumstances, the heart muscle that is fed by the partially blocked vessel receives enough blood under resting conditions (when you're not exercising) and therefore is able to continue working without being damaged.

When you exercise, however, your heart has to work harder in order to pump more blood to the other parts of your body, giving them energy to exercise. In order to do this extra work, your heart requires a greater supply of oxygen and energy. Your body supplies these nutrients to your heart by increasing the blood flow to the heart muscle three- to fivefold via your coronary arteries. If a significant blockage (about 70 to 95 percent) is present in one of the coronary arteries, blood flow can't be increased enough, and that part of the heart doesn't have the necessary energy to perform its duty (pumping blood to the rest of the body). This inadequate supply of blood flow causes the heart muscle to experience distress and you feel pain. This is exactly the point at which Michael began to feel discomfort in his chest.

Once Michael got off the treadmill, he began to feel better almost immediately.

This is because, when you stop exercising and your body no longer requires the extra supply of blood, your heart can return to a resting state, so its need for extra energy decreases. The pain or discomfort or pressure typically dissipates within a few minutes after you stop exercising.

If the pain continues or does not go away at all, you may be experiencing a heart attack, and you should seek medical attention *immediately.* In addition, if you feel pain in your chest when you exercise, don't ignore it simply because it goes away when you stop exerting yourself. It is your body waving a red flag, telling you to seek medical attention immediately!

THE NITTY GRITTY

We explained that in most circumstances a partial blockage will allow the heart to receive the blood supply it requires while at rest. However, if you have many blockages over a period of time, the heart muscle may, in fact, not receive enough blood to continue functioning healthily. It is therefore important to have regular medical care so that problems can be diagnosed and treated as early as possible.

This vigilance about your health is particularly important if you haven't exercised for a while but plan to do so. See your medical practitioner for a checkup before beginning an exercise routine. In addition, other red-flag symptoms that you may experience when you exercise include difficulty breathing while exercising (with or without chest pain, especially if you've never felt this before), chest heaviness or tightness, and tightness in your jaw, neck, or arm. Of course, feeling short of breath may just be a sign that you're not in shape, but you should check it out medically just to be sure, especially if you are really winded.

It is important to note that when you have a partial coronary blockage, you will likely experience chest pain almost every time you exert yourself to a certain degree. However, it is possible that the experience can differ each time, depending on the effort you exert. Sometimes you may have discomfort and at other times you might not. Even if your symptoms are somewhat erratic, make sure you see a doctor.

QUESTION 4

Reginald (75) and his wife, Ida, had been arguing about money, a topic that causes him a great deal of stress and sends his already elevated blood pressure through the roof! Reginald noticed that sometimes, when an argument became really bad, he started to feel a heavy pressure in his chest and sometimes also became light-headed. At first, Reginald thought it was related to smoking (he always chain smoked during an argument). So about two months ago he quit cold turkey. It didn't work. Even without smoking, when he and Ida began to bicker, the symptoms returned. Being calm—not easy when you're in the middle of a fight— is the only way he has found to stop these frightening symptoms from developing or worsening. Therefore, Reginald has been avoiding arguments with Ida at all costs. He's relieved that he has not felt the chest pressure or light-headedness for a while, but he can't help wondering . . .

I think I'm feeling better.
Can I wait a little while before seeing my doctor?

THE BOTTOM LINE

When you are able to avoid symptoms by changing your behavior, it could make you feel better for the moment. You are probably hopeful that this means that you do not have a serious medical condition. However, the truth is actually quite different.

You need to see your doctor as soon as possible!

As we learned in Question 3, a significant blockage in a coronary artery (70 percent or above) can cause chest discomfort and short-ness of breath when you exert yourself but not when you are at rest. Exertion can be exercise, but it also refers to intensely emotional sit-uations (positive or negative), because these also cause your body to increase adrenaline production, requiring your heart to work harder. Some examples of exertion other than exercise include

- A stressful work environment or job loss/change
- Planning or celebrating a significant event, like a wedding or birth
- Arguments (like those between Reginald and Ida)
- Relationship problems
- Financial concerns (exactly what Reginald and Ida argued about)
- Health worries
- Death of a loved one

These, along with exercise, are the main causes of chest discom-fort related to your heart. Of course, depending on your lifestyle, there could be many others. You should be aware that not every chest pain is caused by a coronary blockage. Emotional stress can also cause chest pain that may be triggered by anxiety or a panic attack. Nevertheless, if you are unsure, it is always best to seek medical treatment to rule out a serious medical condition.

These types of stressors typically cause intermittent or occasional chest discomfort. Since people are especially likely to avoid situa-tions that are potentially scary or unpleasant, you may—without realizing it—begin avoiding the stressor in order to avoid the worry associated with the symptoms. It is sort of like refusing to get on the scale because you don't want to know how much you weigh. Reginald avoided discomfort by refusing to argue with his wife. Other people learn exactly how far they can push themselves on a treadmill or a tennis court before they will feel uncomfortable. They may only feel it when they are forced to exert themselves, like when running to catch a bus.

However, the symptoms you are avoiding are actually a red flag that you should not ignore. Your body is asking you to pay attention because something is not right. When you take these symptoms seriously and you see a cardiologist, it is possible that you will be diagnosed with *coronary artery disease* (CAD). CAD is the medical terminology used to describe the plaque buildup in your coronary arteries (see Figure 2). If you have CAD, *diagnosing it in a timely fashion can actually save your life!* Left untreated, CAD can worsen, resulting in more blockages and even a heart attack.

As you may recall, we discussed that heart attacks are most frequently triggered by less significant blockages (those below 70 percent), which don't cause any symptoms. You may, therefore, be wondering why you would be at risk for a heart attack if you *do* have symptoms. The answer is simple: 20 to 30 percent of heart attacks actually occur at the site of an artery that is more than 70 percent blocked. In addition, if you have one blocked artery that is causing you to have symptoms of chest pain, it is virtually certain that this is merely the tip of the iceberg. Once you have a critical blockage (more than 70 percent), this is an indicator that you already have plaque buildup that is causing less severe blockages in virtually *all* of your coronary arteries and therefore significantly increases your chances of having a heart attack. This is why it is critical to pay attention to the warning signs you feel when you exert yourself.

Okay, so you admit that you have been ignoring the warning signs.
Now, how do you know if it's really, really serious?

There are *five* signs that may indicate you have an unstable block-age that could be getting rapidly worse, putting you at risk of an imminent heart attack. If you experience any of these signs, see your doctor right away.

1. Pressure in your chest, shortness of breath, or any other symp-toms you have been experiencing that are *now developing more quickly with exertion* or at a lower intensity than they had before. Reginald noticed that his symptoms started to occur at times other than during an argument. After a while they seemed to appear with very little provocation—a long wait at the super-market checkout, someone cutting him off on the highway, or even while cheering for his favorite sports team.
2. You start to feel symptoms with only minimal activity or with regular, daily exertion.
3. Once the symptoms start, they take longer and longer to resolve.
4. The symptoms *do not* resolve at all after you stopped exercis-ing. If this happens, you may be having a heart attack and you should call 911 immediately.
5. You develop chest pain or shortness of breath *at rest,* without any activity. This could also be a sign that you are having a heart attack. Call 911 immediately.

The good news is that if CAD is treated with the correct medi-cation (chapter 5) and possibly with angioplasty, and if you make appropriate lifestyle changes (chapter 6), your risk of a heart attack in the future is significantly reduced.

THE NITTY GRITTY

After you have been diagnosed with CAD, your physician may then diagnose you with *chronic angina*. Another term for this is *angina pectoris*. *Angina* means "tightness," and *pectoris* means "chest." A diagnosis of chronic angina means that you still have symptoms even after you have been treated with medication or even had an intervention such as stent or bypass surgery.

The reason you may still be symptomatic after treatment is that you may have many blocked blood vessels, some of which may not be treatable with a stent or with bypass surgery, particularly if they are very small blood vessels. Some people find that the symptoms of angina don't trouble them very much, so they elect to treat them with medication alone. Interestingly, about 10 to 30 percent[2, 3] of people who have received a stent or had bypass surgery still experience symptoms of angina.

If you experience angina, you're not alone! It is estimated that about 10 million Americans have chronic angina, with another 500,000 new cases reported each year.[4] Of these, 320,000 are men and 180,000 women. The average number of angina episodes you can expect to experience is reported to be about two a week.

If you do not have any symptoms of angina, does that mean you do not have CAD?

No, not necessarily. It is possible to have significant CAD and even have multiple blockages that are greater than 70 percent without having symptoms of angina. In many cases, people who have silent CAD are very sedentary, and the reason that they do not develop symptoms is because they do not exert themselves enough to challenge their heart muscle. In other instances, a person may have diabetes or another disease that decreases their pain perception. Last, some people may have atypical symptoms (like the ones described in Question 1), which they do not identify as serious.

Q U E S T I O N **5**

At a recent checkup, Diane's (63) doctor suggested that she might have CAD. Although Diane doesn't have any symptoms, she does have three very significant risk factors for heart disease. The first is that her mother died of a massive heart attack at fifty-two years old. Second, Diane has diabetes. And third, Diane is a smoker.

Diane's doctor, who is appropriately conservative, is concerned that Diane may not develop any symptoms of chest pain only because she does not exert herself much. She has chronic back pain, resulting from herniated disks. She underwent back surgery three years ago, and now she has trouble walking even short distances.

Diane is very upset about the possible diagnosis of CAD.

"I don't understand why you would think I have something so bad! I'm not overweight and I don't have high cholesterol!"

"Let's talk for a few minutes," responded the doctor. "It is upsetting to think that you could have heart disease, but don't you think it would be much worse to ignore the red flags and have a heart attack?"

"I guess you're right," said Diane with a sigh, still frustrated and thinking to herself . . .

How did I get this?

THE BOTTOM LINE

After talking with her doctor, Diane discovered that being over-weight and having elevated cholesterol levels are only two possible factors that may put someone at risk for developing plaque deposits in the blood vessels and leading to CAD. She also learned that, in addition to the heart, plaque can affect blood vessels in other parts of the body. When this happens, it is called *peripheral arterial disease* (PAD). PAD can cause leg pain when walking or even a stroke. Blood vessels that may be impacted by peripheral arterial disease include carotid arteries (which are in the neck and supply blood to the brain). Blocked carotid arteries have the potential to cause a stroke. Blocked renal arteries (which are in the kidneys) contribute to high blood pressure or even kidney damage. Last, when the blood vessels in the legs are blocked, it can cause leg pain while walking or even at rest (if the blockages are severe).

The risk factors for CAD and for PAD are similar. Therefore, if you control your risk factors, you will be doing so for both CAD and PAD.

What are the risk factors?

There are actually *five* major risk factors, each of which could lead to CAD or PAD.

1. *Genetics* may be the culprit. If you have a parent, sibling, or child who either had a heart attack or had angioplasty or bypass surgery at a younger age, you may be at risk as well.

   Diane recognized that she had this risk factor. Her mother's heart attack at an early age puts her at risk for a heart attack too.

2. *Smoking* is not just a bad habit that can cause lung cancer, it can increase your risk for a number of diseases, including heart attacks and stroke. In fact, it is statistically more likely that a smoker will develop CAD than die of lung cancer! Clearly, this is the most easily controlled risk factor. If you stop smoking, your risk will be dramatically decreased.

3. *Diabetes* is a major risk factor. In particular, uncontrolled diabetes will substantially increase your risk for CAD and PAD over time. Therefore, if you are diabetic, it is essential that you control your blood sugar levels as much as possible.

Diane now realizes that diabetes has put her at risk for CAD.

4. *High cholesterol* can be a trigger for CAD. Often, people don't know if they have high cholesterol. If you're not sure, ask your doctor to test your blood and review the results with you. If your cholesterol is higher than acceptable limits, you will need to change your eating habits (see question 33). Your doctor may also recommend that you begin taking a cholesterol-lowering medication.

Diane's doctor shared with her that her cholesterol is within acceptable limits. He cautioned Diane to stay vigilant about keeping her weight and cholesterol in a healthy range.

5. *High blood pressure* is a lesser-known cause of CAD, and as with cholesterol, many people rarely check their blood pressure. You don't even have to see your doctor to check your blood pressure. You can do so at almost any drugstore or fire station! But if you discover that your blood pressure is elevated, make an appointment with your doctor in order to get a complete diagnosis and the correct medical treatment.

If, like Diane, you have no symptoms but have any of the risk factors that could lead to CAD and PAD, this is an excellent time to see your doctor to discuss what you should be doing to reduce your overall risk. The key to preventing CAD/PAD (or to slow their progression) and reducing your risk of having a heart attack or stroke is *making the necessary lifestyle changes* that will control your risk factors for CAD.

For now, keep in mind that a sedentary lifestyle and too much processed foods are the primary causes for Type 2 diabetes, high cholesterol, and high blood pressure—three of the five risk factors! But don't worry, in chapters 5 and 6 we will discuss ways that you can reduce your risk factors for developing CAD/PAD.

THE NITTY GRITTY

You're probably wondering exactly how each of the five risk factors could have a direct impact on the health of your heart and the rest of your body.

You are *genetically* at risk if you have at least one first-degree relative who has been diagnosed with CAD or experienced a heart attack at a young age. First-degree relatives include parents, siblings, or children. For it to be a genetic risk factor, the relative must be diagnosed before the age of fifty-five for men and before sixty-five for women. This does not guarantee that you will develop the disease, but it increases the likelihood that you will. Unfortunately, there is no cure for bad genes. However, by making sure you control *all* the other risk factors, you will substantially decrease the risk of developing the disease yourself. Diane's mom's heart attack at fifty-two puts Diane at a genetic risk for having a heart attack.

If you *smoke,* this is the first risk factor you should seek to control. Heart attacks in individuals below the age of fifty almost always occur in smokers. But why does smoking cause CAD and heart attacks? You may not realize it, but smoking is highly destructive to your blood vessels.

Each blood vessel has three layers. The most important, the innermost layer—the endothelium—is a single layer of cells, crucial to maintaining the health of the vessel itself. It is so important that some people consider the one trillion cells that make up the endothelium to be the body's largest organ (it's larger than the liver). The cells of the endothelium act much as Teflon does in a frying pan: they prevent the blood from sticking to the inner lining of the blood vessel as it passes through. Smoking severely damages endothelial cells, causing them to lose their Teflon-like ability and increasing the chance that you will develop blockages.

Diabetes also runs in families, which means that it has a genetic component. However, diabetes can be exacerbated by a less healthy diet, by lack of exercise, and by being overweight. A recent study showed that people with Type 2 diabetes who were able to reduce their body weight through diet and exercise by 7 percent had much better control over their diabetes. In fact, one-third of them were able to stop taking their diabetes medication.[5] Clearly, lifestyle changes are a key factor in controlling diabetes, which will reduce the risk for heart attacks and stroke! We will discuss these lifestyle changes in greater depth in chapter 5. Although Diane doesn't have high cholesterol, her mother did. This means that Diane is at risk for developing high cholesterol too.

If you have been diagnosed with *high cholesterol,* it is important to know that cholesterol—which is part of your blood—actually consists of several different parts. The two most important are LDL (low-density lipoprotein), which is harmful to your body, and HDL (high-density lipoprotein), which is protective. The total cholesterol (which is a combination of LDL, HDL, and some other particles) is actually not nearly as important as knowing your LDL and HDL as separate numbers.

In healthy individuals, LDL cholesterol should be less than 130 mg/dl, but in those diagnosed with CAD we aim for levels below 100 mg/dl (ideally around 70 mg/dl). This can rarely be achieved by diet alone, so medication is often added to achieve these levels. *Statins* are the group of medications commonly used for this purpose. We will talk more about statins as well as other information about LDL in chapters 3 and 5.

In addition to lowering your LDL if it is too high, it is important to *raise* your HDL if it is too low. HDL is responsible for taking cholesterol out of the blood and transporting it back to the liver. HDL thus plays an important role in minimizing the amount of cholesterol plaque deposited, and it even helps to reduce plaque size. Unfortunately, there is little you can do to raise your HDL levels. HDL can be moderately increased by exercising and by drinking no more than one alcoholic beverage a day. There are medications to address HDL, but these are much less effective than the statins are in reducing LDL. Ongoing research is testing newly developed medications that may successfully raise HDL levels, but the results of these studies are still some time away.

Blood pressure, like cholesterol, can be negatively impacted by an unhealthy lifestyle. Sedentary and overweight people are at greatest risk for developing *high blood pressure.* There are some natural ways to reduce blood pressure (see chapters 3 and 5), including exercise, maintaining a healthy body weight, and minimizing salt intake. In addition, many people need to take medication in order to lower and stabilize their blood pressure. It is important to have blood pressure that is successfully controlled, because high blood pressure is a substantial risk factor for heart attacks and an even greater risk factor for stroke.

Now that you understand how and why you may have heart disease, chapter 2 will teach you everything you need to know about the ways in which your cardiologist will evaluate your heart in order to learn more about the symptoms you are experiencing. This is an important step toward making the correct diagnosis and offering you the best possible treatment.

CHAPTER

Two

The Next Steps: Learning More About My Heart

QUESTION **6** ──────────

Reginald was convinced that there was really nothing wrong with him other than a bit of stress caused by a rough patch in his marriage. In fact, he didn't even tell Ida about his symptoms. One day, however, he mentioned the chest pressure to his friend Marcus, who told him that he should see a doctor right away!

The doctor wasn't as unconcerned about the symptoms as Reginald. In fact, she expressed concern that they might mean he has coronary artery disease. In order to be sure, she referred Reginald to a cardiologist to have a stress test. Reginald is worried—now he'll have to tell Ida. In addition, he wants to make sure he gets the right care. The question at the top of his mind is . . .

My family doctor gave me a list of cardiologists. How do I know which one is the best one for me?

THE BOTTOM LINE

Choosing the right cardiologist is an important decision because, if you have heart disease requiring intervention, your cardiologist will become an important part of your life. A relationship with a doctor whom you trust and like will make it easier for you to feel confident when you need to make important decisions about your health.

There is no "one" perfect doctor. Rather, there are cardiologists who will be a better match for your needs and personality. There are several ways to ensure that your search is successful.

Just as you would do with any important project, you will need to do some research to find the right cardiologist. Start with the name or names given to you by your internist or family doctor, but don't stop there. Add to this list the names of doctors given to you by people who have had positive experiences with their cardiologist. In addition, compile a list (hopefully a short one) of doctors whom people do not recommend. Be sure to inquire what they did not like about a particular cardiologist to make sure their gripe isn't petty or personal.

Another way to add names to your list is to do research on the Internet. You can usually read a doctor's bio on the website of hospitals with which they are affiliated, and some doctors have their own websites as well. While Internet research won't necessarily help you learn whether or not you like a doctor, you will be able to learn about his or her affiliations and experience.

Once you have compiled a list of recommended doctors, don't forget to consider proximity to your home. It may be fine and even worthwhile to travel a distance to see a doctor for a first or second opinion, but the one you ultimately choose as *your* physician should have an office close enough to your home that it is not a burden to travel there as frequently as may be necessary. If keeping appointments with a cardiologist feels like a burden because of traffic, trouble parking, or difficulty getting a bus, you will be less likely to see your doctor as often as you might need.

How do I pick the best cardiologist for me?

Of course, your top priority is making sure that your doctor has as much experience as possible. For the most part you will be able to learn this by asking the person who referred you. If you can't find out, you can call the office of each cardiologist you are considering and request that the office manager or nurse tell you about the doctor's background and experience. It is a good sign if the doctor's staff is friendly, open, and willing to talk to you.

Once you have narrowed down your list even more, it is time to make an appointment—or more than one. Whenever possible, it is a good idea to meet at least two doctors. By interviewing multiple physicians, you might learn that there is more than one acceptable method to treat your heart disease. While this may leave you with more questions than answers, it is *always* important to be well informed about your health. These meetings will also help you learn if the doctor relates to you in a way that feels comfortable.

When Reginald told Ida about his symptoms and about the doctor's recommendation to see a cardiologist, at first she was upset that he hadn't told her sooner. But then she jumped into action and began researching cardiologists for him. Before long, Ida's research uncovered two names that kept coming up as the best cardiologists in the area. She made an appointment with one of them.

If you feel that it is important to thoroughly understand the doctor's recommendations and treatment plan, you will want a doctor who can talk to you in plain English and who is willing to clarify and explain your situation until you understand what's going on. Some people don't require this kind of explanation. If you fit into this category, you will not necessarily need a doctor with a perfect bedside manner. Remember, there is no right or wrong. There are many different types of doctors just as there are many different kinds of patients. The key is to find a doctor you can respect and whom you believe respects you.

After meeting the first doctor, Reginald was ready to sign on the dotted line, but Ida wasn't. She didn't think that his explanations were sufficiently clear. In addition, to her, he seemed impatient with her questions. Ida wanted to interview the second doctor. Reginald was fine with this. He was still too nervous and overwhelmed to ask questions. Ida may be the one he fights with, but she's also the one he trusts to take care of him.

In addition to finding a doctor who cares about your experience while in his or her care, it is ideal to find one who keeps up with the latest research and diagnostic and treatment methods within the field. This means that your doctor will be sure to order enough tests and procedures to aid in your diagnosis and treatment but not request unnecessary evaluative procedures. You should ask your doctor to tell you the reason he is ordering each test, what the anticipated outcome will be, and how this result might impact your treatment options. If it appears that a test is being ordered to rule out a very unlikely diagnosis or simply to round out a panel of tests, you are within your rights to refuse the test or to request a second opinion as to whether you really need it.

The second doctor fit the bill for Reginald and Ida! He was knowledgeable, kind, and patient. Both Reginald and Ida believed that he was the best choice.

THE NITTY GRITTY

It is always important to take as much responsibility as you can for your health, and this includes making sure that you are seeing a doctor who is the best match for you. As we have discussed, there are many ways to select the right doctor, including online research. However, it is important to note that some information you find on the Internet can be less useful than you think, and some of it may even be misleading. For example, websites that post reviews of doctors sometimes have only a small number of reviews of a particular physician who may or may not be accurate. As with many online review sites, some people are motivated to post only because they had a fantastic experience (or are a friend or relative of the doctor) or because they had a terrible experience that may or may not have been the doctor's fault (or they are a friend or relative of a competitor). If a review site does not have several reviews of a physician—at least twenty or more—it is likely not a great research source.

More helpful physician ratings might be those based on peer recommendation. This means that other doctors in the area have recommended a particular physician be given a top rating or added to a list of recommended doctors. Of course, it pays not to make this your only criterion for selecting a physician, because some doctors might be popular but not necessarily have top-notch skills.

Another interesting way to research a doctor is to search for his or her name in Google Scholar (http://www.scholar.google.com) or in PubMed (http://www.ncbi.nlm.nih.gov/pubmed). These websites tell you whether a doctor has published in his or her area of expertise. Of course, there are many excellent doctors who do not do research and therefore are not published. Nevertheless, when a doctor regularly publishes research, it ensures that he or she is aware of the newest guidelines and therapies and is also likely to attend the major annual cardiology conferences in order to stay current in the field.

Now that you know how to choose the right cardiologist for you, we will devote the rest of this chapter to the evaluation methods used to determine the health of your heart. This evaluation is the first step your cardiologist will take in caring for you.

QUESTION 7 ————————————

Michael had all but convinced himself that his new exercise regimen was causing him to have a heart attack. When he told his oldest daughter, Jessica, she laughed.

"Dad, you just don't want to exercise. Believe me, it's nothing!"

But Michael continued to worry, because he felt worse every time he walked on the treadmill. Ignoring his family's laughter and jokes, he went to see a cardiologist. The doctor didn't think Michael's symptoms were funny at all. In fact, she recommended that Michael have a stress test in order to be accurately diagnosed.

The doctor explained that the stress test would require Michael to walk on a treadmill in the doctor's office, but that was about all she said. Michael is nervous about whether his symptoms will prevent him from being able to complete the test. In addition, his doctor explained that, because he is having such significant symptoms, she wants to conduct a nuclear study, which is a more sophisticated stress test that includes imaging. Michael's mind is swimming with all the details, but his main question is . . .

My cardiologist just told me to get a stress test. What does that mean?

THE BOTTOM LINE

A doctor will typically order a stress test when she is concerned that you may have one or more critical blockages in your coronary arteries. Usually, a doctor will order a stress test if someone is experiencing chest discomfort or other symptoms when he exercises or experiences emotional stress. These symptoms signal the strong possibility of a serious blockage, which can then be confirmed with the stress test. In most cases, a stress test simulates an exercise environment, which is where the treadmill fits in. This is because the symptoms typically occur when a person exerts himself.

What is a stress test?

A stress test is usually performed in the cardiologist's office or at a hospital under the supervision of a trained nurse, an exercise physiologist, and a medical doctor. Stress tests are considered very safe. They are associated with a less than 0.01 percent mortality and less than 0.05 morbidity.[6] But it is still important for them to be performed with adequate supervision. In most cases, your doctor will not perform the actual stress test. This is the job of a nurse and a technician. Also, these professionals may not all be in the room with you throughout the test, but at least one of them will be there to assist you in case you don't feel well. In fact, a medical doctor is readily available in the office in case of an emergency, even if you don't see your doctor during the procedure. Michael was relieved to hear this!

You should not eat or smoke for at least three hours prior to the test. You should also avoid caffeinated beverages for three hours before a regular stress test and for twelve hours before a test with medication (see Question 8 for more discussion about this). You should continue taking medications unless your doctor instructs otherwise. If you're not sure, ask your doctor a few days before your stress test. You should also refrain from exercising just before the test.

You should arrive at the appointment in comfortable shoes and loose-fitting clothing. Before beginning the test, the nurse or technician will adhere electrodes to several places on your chest (electrodes are little stickers). This does not hurt. The wires attached to the electrodes are connected to an EKG machine that will continuously record the electrical waves of your heart as well as your heart rate during the stress test. Subtle changes on the EKG during the test may indicate that a part of your heart is receiving inadequate blood supply as a result of a blocked artery. In addition, your blood pressure will be checked at regular intervals.

In most cases, a stress test will require you to walk on a treadmill that will gradually increase in speed and elevation every two minutes. (See Question 8 if you cannot walk on a treadmill.) You should try to walk on the treadmill for as long as possible. The longer you can endure, the better the test result will be! Most people will need to stop walking because of fatigue, leg pain, shortness of breath, or chest pain. If, during the stress test, your body produces the symptoms that you experience with your usual exertion, this is helpful in confirming a diagnosis. However, if you don't feel any symptoms before the end of the test, don't worry. It doesn't mean the test was inadequate. In some cases, the test is terminated even though you feel you could have pushed yourself further. This is usually the case, because you have reached your *target heart rate,* also known as the optimal heart rate during exercise, which is a predetermined number based on your age.

How accurate is a stress test?

It is important to realize that stress tests are not 100 percent accurate. This is because there is a small chance that a blockage is present that isn't picked up by the test (called a false negative) or that the stress test results are abnormal—you "fail" the test although there is no significant blockage (called a false positive). Women are more likely to have false positive results than men, so some cardiologists believe that women should have a stress test that includes imaging, because it is more accurate (more about imaging below in the Nitty Gritty section). Michael's doctor, however, ordered a test with imaging because, given Michael's symptoms, the doctor wanted the most accurate diagnosis possible.

In addition to a small number of false negatives and false positives, remember that a stress test (like other exercise and exertion) will only cause you to have symptoms if you have a severe blockage *greater than 70 percent* (review chapter 1 for more information on this). Therefore, passing a stress test does *not* rule out the possibility that you may have mild to moderate CAD—plaque buildup with blockages of less than 70 percent. As you may recall from chapter 1, less severe blockages do not cause you to become symptomatic, because they continue to allow enough blood to flow to the heart muscle, even during exertion. It is therefore possible, although unlikely, to have a normal stress test and still have a heart attack shortly thereafter. Most heart attacks are caused by blockages of *less than* 70 percent. A stress test can only detect blockages that are severe enough to cause symptoms like exertional angina. It is important to understand that the stress test *cannot* detect CAD in the absence of symptoms, because it will almost always miss *all* less severe blockages.

In addition to confirming or rejecting the possibility that your chest pain is due to a blockage, a stress test can also help determine the amount of CAD you may have, because if you have one or more significant blockages (more than 70 percent blocked) you may have *many* minor blockages. A major blockage is almost always the tip of the iceberg. On the other hand, if the stress test is normal (no critical blockage), it is possible that you have a few noncritical blockages, but probably many fewer than if you also had a critical blockage. In this scenario, your risk of a heart attack is lower than if you have a critical blockage and many less critical blockages.

Michael's stress test was not normal. In fact, it indicated a strong likelihood that he had significant CAD, which would require further diagnosis and treatment. Needless to say, when Jessica found out that her dad probably had heart disease, she felt awful that she had made fun of him. She was also glad that he had ignored her and had seen a doctor.

THE NITTY GRITTY

There are two different ways of performing a stress test. The simplest stress test is with an EKG alone, as we discussed above. While this is a relatively easy test to perform and should take less than a half hour, the EKG waves are not always accurate in picking up blockages, because as we pointed out earlier, there are times when the test produces false positives and false negatives. In fact, there is an approximately 30 percent error rate on both sides, resulting in both false positives and false negatives. Therefore, in order to make the test more accurate, your doctor may order a stress test with imaging, which means that pictures are taken of your heart while you exercise. A stress test with imaging is more accurate. It decreases the chances of false negatives and false positives to about 10 to 20 percent. The downside of this test is that imaging of the heart is achieved by injection of a low dose of radioactive nuclear material, which exposes a person to some radiation. The dose of radiation is similar to that received during a whole body CT scan, or, on average, about four to five times as much as the radiation to which a person is exposed due to radiation from the earth and the atmosphere (known as background radiation[7]).

This test is more accurate because the injected material can outline the location in the heart muscle that is affected by the blockage. A healthy heart will pump the nuclear material evenly throughout the heart muscle. However, when there is a blockage, the part of the heart muscle that is supplied by the blocked artery will receive less blood during exercise and will therefore receive less of the nuclear material. Directly after the stress test, a camera able to detect the radiation from the nuclear material is used to take pictures of your heart. Any differences in the distribution of the nuclear material will be detected and the location of blockages can be determined.

It is possible to improve the sensitivity and accuracy of a regular EKG stress test without exposure to radiation. One option is an ultrasound of the heart (echocardiogram) in conjunction with the stress test. This technique is not as commonly prescribed as the test that requires an injection of radioactive materials. An ultrasound requires a high level of expertise, thus its accuracy is somewhat dependent on the skill level of the technician. Your doctor will determine which of the three stress tests is best for you, and this recommendation will be determined by many factors. You should discuss the potential alternatives with your doctor and make sure you understand why a particular test is ordered.

In addition to determining whether you have critical blockages, a stress test also offers information about your general fitness level, which can determine how healthy you may be in the future. The measure of a person's fitness, as determined by a stress test, is called *maximal work capacity* or *peak functional capacity*. This measure is calculated by the amount of time and the level of intensity at which you exercised during the test. Simply speaking, the faster and longer you endure, the better your fitness level, and the better your fitness level, the greater your prognosis for long-term health and survival.

QUESTION 8

After speaking with her primary care doctor about her risk factors for heart disease, Diane agreed to see a cardiologist. At the end of her first visit, the cardiologist strongly recommended that she have a stress test. She explained to Diane that a stress test involved walking on a treadmill. When Diane heard this, she was immediately concerned that, due to her back injury, walking on the treadmill would be much too painful for her, so she asked her doctor . . .

I can't walk on a treadmill. Can I still take a stress test?

THE BOTTOM LINE

Diane's doctor assured her that she could still have the stress test. In fact, Diane is not alone. Many people are not able to walk on a treadmill due to back injuries, back pain, or for many other reasons. Nevertheless, even with this limitation, it is still important to determine whether you have critical coronary blockages. The doctor is able to simulate the stress test's effect on your heart with the use of intravenous (IV) medications. This test, which involves no exercise at all, is called a *pharmacologic stress test*. One of two types of medications is used to trick your heart into an exercise state. One medication increases blood flow in the heart and the other increases heart rate. Since both of these mechanisms occur with exercise, the medications imitate the experience of exercising.

So what will I have to do?

First, you will be asked to lie down on an examination table. You will not be required to do any physical activity. An IV needle will be placed in your arm, and the medication will be administered through the IV. Once the medication begins to work, you may experience chest discomfort (usually a burning sensation) and shortness of breath. It's not unusual to experience significant discomfort that makes you panic or think that you are having a heart attack. In truth, these symptoms are benign and transient, typically lasting only a few minutes.

Knowing about these potential symptoms in advance will alleviate your anxiety and make it easier for you to take the test. It is also comforting to know that your vital signs will be closely monitored throughout the pharmacologic stress test.

Diane was nervous, but her understanding of what to expect helped reduce her anxiety. She also brought her best friend, Evelyn, with her to the stress test. Although Evelyn could not accompany her into the evaluation, just knowing that she was in the waiting room was comforting for Diane.

In order to view the results of a pharmacologic stress test, it must be conducted in conjunction with one of the two types of imaging studies that we discussed in Question 7.

I can walk a little, but it seems so much easier to do the pharmacologic test. Should I just do that?

Actually, no. It is always better to exercise if you are able to do so. Patients sometimes choose a pharmacologic test because they are afraid that they won't be able to exercise long enough to be able to complete the traditional treadmill stress test. In fact, even if you can't exercise for very long, this test provides your doctor with important information about your health and even your future health. The information that your doctor learns by calculating your endurance can help him guide you toward making lifestyle changes that will impact your quality of life over the next several years. So don't be afraid to try the exercise stress test. If you can't reach your target heart rate (which determines if the stress test is of good enough quality to provide meaningful results), your doctor can easily complement this test with a medication stress test in order to achieve the necessary results.

THE NITTY GRITTY

As you have just learned, a pharmacologic stress test is performed using one of two types of medications, and it is accompanied by an imaging evaluation. The medication your doctor chooses will depend upon which type of imaging will be used. If your doctor chooses a nuclear stress test (using radioactive nuclear material) for imaging, the medication will need to increase blood flow to the heart in order to move the radioactive materials into and around the heart muscle. The medications that perform this action are Persantine, Adenosine, and Regadenoson. One of these will be used for your stress test. The increased blood flow, triggered by the medication, will cause the nuclear material to distribute unevenly in the presence of a blockage.

The area fed by the blockage will receive less of the nuclear material. This *differential uptake* will be determined by imaging the heart with a nuclear camera.

It is important to note that these medications can cause intense chest discomfort during the test because they directly activate and stimulate the nerve endings in your chest. Although this may sound feel scary, there is actually nothing dangerous happening to your chest or heart. In addition, you will be very closely monitored at all times. Fortunately, this uncomfortable feeling lasts only a few minutes and can actually be reversed with another medication after the stress test is complete.

When your doctor decides to use ultrasound imaging (echocardiogram), the medication of choice is dubutamine (thus the procedure is called a dobutamine stress echocardiogram). Dobutamine will increase your heart rate and the squeezing function of your heart, closely mimicking exercise conditions.

You will receive an ultrasound (echocardiogram) so your doctor can see how your heart functions at baseline, prior to the medication infusion. Then another ultrasound will be conducted during the infusion to observe how your heart functions when stressed.

During the infusion, you may feel your heart racing or you might experience some palpitations. Chest pain, another side effect, is much less common. As with the medications used in a nuclear stress test, this medication also has a short half-life. So once the infusion is over, any symptoms you might experience will resolve quickly.

During the test, if you do not have a blockage, all parts of the heart muscle will move with similar vigor. However, in the presence of a blockage, some areas of the heart will receive a decreased blood supply when the Dobutamine infusion increases the heart's workload. These areas will squeeze less vigorously when compared to the areas that have an adequate supply of blood. The difference in blood flow will be detected when the doctor looks at the images of your heart with the echocardiogram.

After the pharmacologic stress test was completed, Diane waited anxiously for four days to get the test results. When she sat down to discuss the results with her doctor, she was still nervous, so she invited Evelyn into the meeting to listen and take notes. It's always good to have more than one set of ears when you meet with your doctor, especially when you are worried. Diane's doctor confirmed that, in fact, she seemed to have a blockage in at least one coronary vessel. Diane was upset but remembered what her internist had told her. It's better to catch it now rather than wait and have a heart attack.

QUESTION 9 _____

After arriving at the ER by ambulance, Brian learned that he was having a heart attack. Fortunately, he received an emergency angioplasty and a stent to open the blockage. Brian's relief that he survived the heart attack was somewhat dampened when his doctor told him that after a heart attack there is frequently some degree of damage to the heart. He learned that after blood flow has been restored to the heart muscle (via the stent) it takes about two to three months for the heart muscle to recover fully, but in some cases it never fully recovers. The doctor explained that it was important to assess Brian's heart to determine its level of functioning. Brian is now wondering . . .

What other tests could my doctor prescribe?

THE BOTTOM LINE

EKG

In addition to a stress test, a few other tests may be used to evaluate your heart. The most basic test is an EKG. In Question 7 we talked briefly about EKGs because of its use during a stress test. In addition to this, an EKG can assess for many cardiac disorders, including the evidence of a prior heart attack. Unlike its use as part of a stress test, a regular EKG is conducted while you are at rest. (No treadmill necessary!) In addition, an EKG takes a sample of only a few seconds of heart activity rather than continuously recording electrical waves while you are moving (as is the case with a stress test). Thus, a regular EKG reflects your heart's performance in a resting state, while a stress-test EKG records changes *over time* throughout the exercise period. The results of an EKG are recorded and printed as wavy lines on a paper that feeds out of the EKG machine.

It is important to note that the EKG is not a very sensitive test, therefore it is not able to detect the presence of many blockages. In fact, in the absence of substantial damage to the heart muscle, a resting EKG can be completely normal, even if there are multiple critical blockages. This is why a stress test is better at determining if critical blockages are present.

Echocardiogram

In addition to an EKG, an echocardiogram or "echo" (also known as a *sonogram* or *ultrasound*) is another commonly ordered test. You may remember that we discussed this test in Questions 7 and 8. During an echocardiogram, images of the heart are recorded and displayed on a monitor. Unlike an EKG, which records the electrical activity of your heart and records this activity on paper, an echocardiogram can display actual images of your heart. The echo is a live test because your doctor can see your heart beating on the screen as it happens (similar to an ultrasound of a fetus).

During this test you will lie on an examination table and a gel will be applied to your chest. This gel helps to form a tight seal between the skin and a transducer. The latter is then pressed against your skin in order to record the images. An echocardiogram is typically painless, although it might feel a bit uncomfortable when pressure is exerted on your chest wall or upper abdomen. This test, which typically takes fifteen to thirty minutes, is mainly used to evaluate the squeezing function of the heart muscle and the heart valves.

When an echocardiogram is conducted on a person who has had a heart attack, it will detect parts of the heart muscle that are not working or that are working below the normal level. This type of finding is a red flag that CAD may be present, which will require further evaluation.

As with an EKG, however, if there is no damage to the heart muscle (that is, no signs of a prior heart attack), an echocardiogram will not pick up coronary artery blockages, even if the blockages are severe. For this reason, an echocardiogram is sometimes combined with a stress test, which is then called a *stress echocardiogram*. We briefly discussed the stress echocardiogram in Question 7.

Three months after Brian's heart attack, his cardiologist requested that Brian have an echocardiogram. The test results indicated that a part of his heart muscle was scarred from the heart attack and was under-performing. Brian's cardiologist explained that this meant that, due to the heart attack, Brian's heart had suffered some damage, despite their opening the blockage with a stent. However, in all likelihood, the damage would have been much more extensive if Brian had not been rushed to the hospital and received the angioplasty procedure quickly.

The amount of blood pumped from the heart into the body (as reflected by the squeezing of the heart muscle) is called *ejection fraction* (EF). A normal EF is 55 to 65 percent.

Brian's EF after his heart attack was 45 percent, which is about a quarter less than the normal 60 percent. Brian was shocked at first. He felt better, though, when his doctor explained that most people can manage satisfactorily with an EF of 45 percent. In fact, because the heart can compensate to a certain extent, people with an EF of 45 percent have minimal or no symptoms at all. We will discuss EF in greater detail in the Nitty Gritty.

Typically, one becomes symptomatic when the heart function is reduced by about a half, meaning an EF of about 30 to 35 percent. But everyone's heart is different, and if your EF is less than 35 percent, you may require further tests or procedures.

In addition to evaluating your heart function, an echocardiogram is able to identify heart valve abnormalities (a cartoon of the heart valves is shown in Figure 4). Blockages or leakages of the heart valves are not the same as blockages of the coronary arteries. Heart valve blockages or leakages can sometimes lead to severe symptoms, like breathing difficulties.

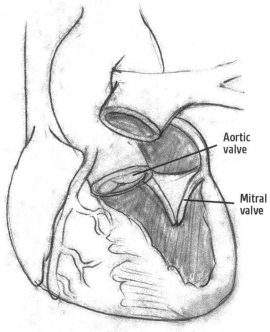

Aortic valve

Mitral valve

Figure 4

CAT scan

A CAT scan also is commonly used to evaluate the heart. CAT scans of the heart have been available for only a few years, but their use is increasing. A CAT scan is noninvasive and can be administered without or more frequently with an x-ray dye (known as *contrast material*). It is primarily used to detect blockages in the coronary arteries.

If a CAT scan detects blockages so easily, why not use it first?

CAT scans are not all that perfect. It is very good at ruling out disease (blockages) in people with healthy coronary arteries, but it is not nearly as proficient at determining the severity of a blockage when there is plaque buildup. This is because the calcifications in the coronary arteries appear as a shadow on the test, and it is sometimes difficult to determine whether the shadow is a severe or only a mild blockage. In addition, a CAT scan exposes you to radiation, especially if it needs to be repeated periodically. Nevertheless, there is ongoing research examining this new technology to determine its best uses in the future.

THE NITTY GRITTY

More about the EKG

In addition to evaluating your heart for critical damage, an EKG has many other uses. It is easily administered in the doctor's office, and its results are immediately available. For these reasons, it is typically the first test ordered by your cardiologist. Brian had his first EKG in the emergency room when he came in complaining about chest pain.

In addition to detecting heart attacks, EKGs are very useful for detecting arrhythmias (*electrical problems with the heart*). Although most electrical problems are unrelated to blockages (*part of the plumbing system*), it is possible for a critical blockage to lead to dangerous arrhythmias, which can be discovered with an EKG.

More about echocardiograms

As you may recall, the difference between a regular echocardiogram and a stress echocardiogram is that a regular echocardiogram evaluates the heart under resting conditions, not while moving on the treadmill or with medication. At rest, unless you have had a heart attack, your echocardiogram will appear normal, even if there are severe blockages of the coronary arteries. However, as you know, during a stress echocardiogram, these blockages can be detected because the heart muscle does not receive an adequate supply of blood while stressed with exercise or medication and will therefore appear weaker on echocardiogram imaging.

What exactly is the EF?

EF refers to the amount of blood (measured in percent) that is ejected from or squeezed out of the left heart cavity (called the *left ventricle*) in a single heartbeat. As we explained above, a normal EF is in the range of 55 to 65 percent. An EF of 60 percent therefore means that 60 percent of the left ventricular blood volume is squeezed out into the body while 40 percent remains in the heart. The reason that the EF cannot be 100 percent is that if all the blood were ejected from the ventricle, there would be a vacuum in the heart. People often become worried when they learn that their heart is working at 60 percent, believing that 100 percent is healthy. They don't realize that, in fact, this number is within the normal range. Now that you know, you won't be upset if you get an excellent result of 60 percent.

More about the CAT scan

As we mentioned above, CAT scans are a fairly new technology for evaluating heart disease. There are two types of CAT scans: one uses an x-ray dye as part of the test, the other is a simpler test and is used primarily to screen for blockages, which we noted as being less accurate in determining the extent of any blockages. This second type of AT scan is used to detect calcifications of the blood vessels but not much more. Calcification occurs when calcium is deposited in the plaque that makes up a blockage. This transforms the blockage into a bonelike structure (which is why it is called "hardening of the arteries"). A CAT scan is only able to detect calcification once a significant amount is deposited into the plaque. It is thus possible to have plaque buildup without the presence of calcifications (known as *soft plaque*), which would be missed a regular CAT scan.

To enable the CAT scan to be more accurate, x-ray (contrast) dye is administered intravenously during the test. The dye allows for visualization of the actual arteries, and most important, it is capable of detecting *both* soft and hard plaque. Two potential shortcomings of a CAT scan with contrast are the exposure to radiation and a risk that the dye could cause kidney damage. Nevertheless, within an expert medical setting, this can offer very accurate results and can sometimes avoid more invasive testing, such as a coronary angiogram (see Question 13).

QUESTION **10** —————————

When the results of Diane's evaluation were returned, she sat down with her doctor to discuss them. After the meeting, Diane was very upset. At times like this she really misses her husband, George, who died five years ago. Fortunately, her friend Evelyn is there to support her when she calls to say . . .

My doctor just gave me my test results. I probably have heart disease. What should I do now?

THE BOTTOM LINE

Diane's doctor explained that her stress test with medication had produced abnormal results, indicating the strong likelihood that she had coronary blockages.

If it turns out that, like Diane, you have multiple risk factors for CAD (see Question 5) or symptoms of CAD (like chest discomfort) in addition to an abnormal stress test, there is a good chance that you have one or more coronary blockages. These red flags indicate a high likelihood that part of your heart is not receiving an adequate blood supply.

Nevertheless, as we have discussed, a stress test does not always yield perfect results. It may produce a false-positive result, meaning that there appears to be a critical blockage but in reality there isn't one. On the other hand, the test can also produce a false-negative or false-normal result, which means that there is a blockage that was not picked up by the stress test.

Keeping in mind these potential inaccuracies, your doctor may recommend further evaluation, even if your stress test did not produce abnormal results. Your doctor may take one of two potential routes. The first possibility is to order a procedure called a *heart catheterization,* also known as a *coronary angiogram.* This is typically requested when the results of a stress test are either abnormal or inconclusive and the suspicion of having blockages is relatively high. Heart catheterization is the best and most accurate test to determine definitively whether you have coronary blockages and, if so, exactly where they are. Briefly during the coronary angiogram an x-ray dye is injected into your heart vessels (coronary arteries), and then pictures are taken of each vessel. This allows your doctor to visualize all the coronary arteries and determine whether there are blockages. (See Question 13 for more details about this procedure.)

The second option your doctor may choose, before ordering any more procedures, is to treat you with medication to see if your chest discomfort or other symptoms are relieved and whether they recur. The determination as to whether you are a candidate for the "take medication and observe" route will depend upon many factors, including

- **Understanding the specific nuances of the stress test.** For example, was there just a small area of the heart that receives less blood or is a larger area involved? If there appears to be significant damage, your doctor may feel more comfortable ordering further evaluation.

  In Diane's case, the damage appeared to be only in a small area.

- **The risk factors.** The larger the number of risk factors you have, the greater your chance of having extensive blockages.

  Diane has many risk factors. She is a smoker, she has diabetes, and she has a family history of heart disease.

- **Your symptoms**. For example, do you experience symptoms with only minimal activity, or does it take a lot of exertion to bring on your symptoms?

  Diane has not had any symptoms of which she is aware.

- **Your comfort level.** Some people feel that they want to know everything that is going on inside their heart as quickly and clearly as possible. Others are willing to take a wait-and-see approach, because they would prefer not to undergo another procedure if they can avoid it. In most instances, even those who are anxious elect to undergo heart catheterization so they can find out for sure whether they have a blockage.

Now that Diane knows something might be wrong, she is too nervous to try medication to see if her symptoms decrease. She wants to have a coronary angiogram so she can have clear information about what is going on inside her body. She also believes that if she learns definitively that she does have blockages, it might motivate her to adopt a healthier lifestyle.

- **Your cardiologist's comfort level.** Most cardiologists believe it is worthwhile to take the *very* small amount of risk associated with the coronary angiogram in order to know exactly how severe the blockages may be and, very important, where they are. Once the test has clearly mapped the blockages, it is easier for your doctor to decide whether treatment should include medicine alone, a stent, or bypass surgery.

Diane's doctor agreed with her that she should have the coronary angiogram. She was particularly concerned about Diane's risk factors in conjunction with the abnormal stress test.

If you and your cardiologist decide that a coronary angiogram is a good idea, your doctor may or may not perform this procedure himself. Highly specialized cardiologists, called *invasive* or *interventional cardiologists*, perform heart catheterizations. Therefore, if your cardiologist does not have this training, he will refer you to an interventional cardiologist within his group of doctors or send you to a doctor who is affiliated with a hospital. As with any other referral, you will want to investigate the doctor's training and experience with this procedure. Of course, if you trust your general cardiologist, it is also important to trust that he will refer you to another good doctor. You might also want to ask how many heart catheterizations are performed annually at the facility where you will have your procedure and inquire about the hospital staff's expertise.

Diane's cardiologist referred her to an interventional cardiologist whom Diane liked very much. Not only did she have the necessary experience and skill level to perform the procedure, she also clearly and thoroughly explained everything to Diane.

THE NITTY GRITTY

Your doctor may recommend a CAT scan of your heart instead of a coronary angiogram. You can refer back to Question 9 for more information about this test. The advantage of a CAT scan is that it is a noninvasive test (unlike the coronary angiogram, no catheters or tubes are placed inside your body), which means that there are almost no inherent risks. This sounds good, but there are only a limited number of medical centers that have the ability to read the results with the high quality necessary for accuracy. In addition, a CAT scan cannot always determine, with precision, the extent of a blockage. Finally, once a CAT scan confirms the very high suspicion of a blockage, you will still need an invasive coronary angiogram to fix the blockage with a stent. For these reasons, a CAT scan is rarely recommended when someone has a high risk for having critical coronary blockages.

Prior to your scheduled procedure, it is important to meet with the interventional cardiologist at the doctor's office or at the hospital. At this meeting, you and the doctor will discuss several issues:

- Your doctor will need to familiarize herself with your general medical condition. Make sure you tell her about *all* the chronic diseases you may have, such as diabetes, chronic obstructive pulmonary disease (COPD), asthma, or rheumatoid arthritis.

Diane remembered to tell her doctor that she has diabetes.

- Once the doctor assesses your general condition, she will be able to determine the best location into which the tube should be inserted to perform the procedure (this is called the *access site*).

Based on Diane's conversation with her interventional cardiologist, the doctor explained that, in her case, the best location to insert the tube was in an artery of her wrist. Diane was surprised, as she did not know that this procedure could be done through her arm. Her doctor explained that, in fact, the more common access site is through a larger artery in the groin area. However, women are at slightly higher risk of bleeding problems when the tube is removed, and by going through the wrist, this risk of bleeding is minimized. In addition, Diane has difficulty lying on her back for a long time because of her herniated disks. By using her wrist, she will be able to sit up immediately after the procedure, which will make it much more comfortable for her.

- Your doctor will evaluate your kidney function. If your kidneys are not working perfectly, the doctor will take precautionary measures to minimize risk of the x-ray dye further harming your kidneys.

- Your doctor will determine which stent may be best for you if, during the procedure, she determines that you require angioplasty. Be sure to tell your doctor if you are not able to take blood thinners (due to an allergy or bleeding problems). This is important, because as you will learn later in the book, there are different types of stents, some of which require you to take blood thinners after you have had the procedure.

Since Diane does not have any complications related to her blood, her doctor is free to choose a stent that requires her to take a blood thinner.

- Tell your doctor if you have any surgical procedure scheduled in the near future. Most surgeons prefer not to operate on a patient who is taking blood thinners. Therefore, if you have angioplasty and receive a stent that requires you to take a blood thinner, it may be difficult for you to have your other surgery. This is because you may not be able to stop taking the blood thinners once the stent has been placed.
- Let your doctor know if your insurance plan does not cover medications. Blood-thinning medications are relatively expensive, so if you need to pay for them yourself, you may want to minimize the amount of time that you need to take them.

QUESTION **11** ───────────

After her heart attack, Rosa has slowly begun to resume her normal activities, but she really has to take it easy. Understandably, Eduardo and their two daughters, Lisa and Donna, are concerned about her health, and they frequently ask Rosa questions about how she is feeling and what's going on with her medically. Even though she knows her family means well, sometimes Rosa becomes overwhelmed with all the questions, and she can't help thinking . . .

My husband and kids ask me questions about what's going on with my heart, but I don't always remember what the doctors told me. How do I get better at that?

THE BOTTOM LINE

When you have a potentially serious health issue, it is normal to feel overwhelmed and stressed. It can be difficult to focus on everything your doctors tell you. It's also challenging to decide which issues you must address immediately and which might be able to wait. For some people, however, the most stressful aspect of learning about a health problem is trying to figure out when and how to convey this information to family and friends.

Some people become annoyed when others ask questions, because it feels like a burden to have to explain a topic you may not yet fully understand. In addition, you may even find it difficult to focus on your doctor's advice and feedback. Other people find it difficult to talk about their heart disease. This is often because talking to friends and family about a serious heart concern makes it feel more real and much scarier. Still other people don't want to burden those closest to them with their medical problems, even when asked.

Despite feelings like these (and any others you may have), it is important to consider the importance of sharing your diagnosis, evaluation, and treatment with those closest to you. To begin, no matter how difficult it may be to discuss your health, it is in your best interest to do so. Sharing the burden of *any* stressful situation almost always alleviates a degree of stress. Since reduced stress is beneficial to both physical and emotional health, anything you can do to alleviate your stress will help your heart!

It is normal if you want to avoid talking to your loved ones about your situation because you don't understand everything that your doctor has explained to you. You don't want to appear naive. Nevertheless, your dilemma makes it even more important for you to get some support from the people who are emotionally close to you. Sometimes other people can ask questions that you didn't or couldn't ask, and they even clarify information for you so that it makes sense. Your friends and family won't feel that your need to discuss your health is a burden on them. In all likelihood, the anxiety of not knowing is much more worrying to them than having the opportunity to help and support you.

You've convinced me!
So what are the best ways to involve my family and friends?

There are several ways to help yourself by inviting those close to you to support you through this stage of your life. At the same time you will alleviate some of their worry about you by giving them a chance to participate in the process.

- **Take someone with you to each medical appointment.** Ask your partner, child, or best friend to attend each appointment with you. Encourage them to participate and to ask questions and take notes. Give all your doctors permission (written if necessary) to talk to your companion freely about your health. This will help you if you are too intimidated or overwhelmed to ask yourself.

  Rosa asked her oldest daughter, Lisa, to go with her to her appointments. Lisa is an organized person who is not afraid to ask questions. In addition, she works from home, so Rosa doesn't feel guilty about asking her to step away from her desk to join her at the doctor. For Rosa, Lisa had all the right qualities for this job.

- **Take notes at every appointment.** If you aren't able to have someone attend each appointment with you, take a notebook and write down everything the doctor says—even things you don't completely understand. Then, after the appointment, review your notes with someone you trust. As you review these notes, you or your confidante may have questions or concerns that you would like the doctor to address. Write these down too. We don't always remember everything that we think we will! You can address them with your doctor by telephone or at your next appointment.

Rosa asked Lisa to do this, and on the rare occasions that Lisa couldn't attend, Rosa took notes herself and shared them with Eduardo and the girls after the appointment.

- **Schedule periodic family meetings.** Often, people have several close family members (like children and grandchildren) in many different places. Each of these people is interested in your health and wants regular updates. It can be tiring to have to explain your situation over and over again. To avoid this, schedule a regular time, as often as you feel comfortable, to have a face-to-face or phone conference with all of them at the same time. Alternatively, you can send an update by email to the whole group, or if you are more comfortable with delegating, you might speak directly to one family member and assign him or her to be in charge of contacting the rest of the family via email or phone.

Lisa created an email group and has kept close family members— Donna, her mom's sister and brother, and the oldest grandchildren—up to date with Rosa's progress.

- **Ask for help with specific issues.** If you need to research doctors, procedures, or treatments, ask someone organized and computer savvy to help you with your research. Not only will it be helpful to you, it will make them feel good to be able to provide you with the help that you need.

Donna is the perfect person for this job. She has free time during the day while her kids are in school, and she is very happy to help her mom learn all there is to know about the procedures the doctor has recommended.

- **Choose one person in whom you can confide about, not only medical information, but also your feelings**. As we mentioned, reduced stress is a very important part of managing your medical health—heart health is negatively impacted by stress. In addition, being able to limit your stress has also been shown to help the process of physical healing. It is therefore important to choose someone to whom you can chat regularly about your worries and fears. Talking about these emotional issues with someone who cares, will definitely help you feel less stressed and upset. Be sure that you choose a confidante who is realistic about the medical issues as well as encouraging and optimistic about your prognosis, because this will be very beneficial to you emotionally.

Rosa talks to Eduardo every day about how she is feeling. On those days that Eddie seems stressed or overwhelmed himself, Rosa calls her best friend, Lydia, who certainly understands what Rosa is experiencing, because her husband had angioplasty two years ago. Since Lydia's husband is doing very well, she is a good, upbeat sounding board for Rosa.

THE NITTY GRITTY

In some situations, a person finds that a health issue doesn't bring out the best in other people, but rather acts as a catalyst to bring out the worst in their close relationships. The appointments, decisions, and emotional turmoil may disrupt an already shaky marriage. A child or best friend's apparent lack of concern can cause you to feel upset and disappointed. In situations like these, it can feel like the rug has truly been pulled out from beneath you, and you don't have anyone to whom you can turn during this stressful time in your life. If this happens to you, you need to do one of two things.

1. **Assess whether there is someone else outside of your immediate circle on whom you can lean.** There are many caring people in the world, so you might be surprised to find that a coworker, cousin, or friend is more than willing to support you at this time. People who have experienced health issues themselves are particularly likely to want to help others. Don't be afraid to reach out. You may find that you have a new best friend before too long!

2. **Seek professional support.** If you are feeling particularly alone, confused, worried, or upset, this may be a good time to meet with a psychologist, social worker, or religious leader for support. A professional can help you develop coping strategies and offer ideas about managing your stress. In addition, this person can be a strong shoulder when you most need one. If you're not sure how to find the right support, speak to one of your doctors for a referral. Your primary care doctor (internist or family doctor) likely has the best access to such a referral.

Some people have the opposite problem: the person closest to you becomes too controlling or bossy and tries to manage your health more than you like. This usually happens when your child or partner is worried about you and tries to take over as a way to manage his or her own anxiety. If you would like your family member or friend to take a step back and let you maintain control of your own health, it is important to say something. Do it in a way that will not lead to hurt on either side. These four steps will help you achieve that goal:

1. Begin by thanking the person for how much he cares about you and your health. Remark how fortunate you feel to have someone so attentive in your life.

2. Explain that while it is important for you to have such great support, you also want to feel like you are remaining in control of the decisions about your health. It can be helpful to explain that it is very difficult to feel that your diagnosis has made you feel that you have lost control of one aspect of your *physical* health—no one chooses heart disease. Therefore, it is important for you to remain in charge of the steps that will bring you as close as possible to being healthy again.

3. Remind the person that you truly value her support and opinions. Explain that you would like her to remain involved in this process as a sounding board and a frequent shoulder to lean on.

4. If, after this conversation, you find the person's behavior doesn't change, you may need to stop sharing information with him in order to control the decisions that you make about your health.

CHAPTER

Three

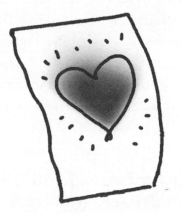

I Just Found Out That
I Have Heart Disease

Michael and his family were upset to learn that his stress test had yielded abnormal results. His daughter Jessica insisted on going with him to the cardiologist to get the results and to learn the treatment recommendations. She thought that it was the least she could do since she had initially underestimated the seriousness of his symptoms. The doctor explained to Michael that there were a few treatment options that may be beneficial to him. The first step that the doctor took was to prescribe several medications for Michael to begin taking immediately.

Michael felt better getting started with treatment immediately, but the first thought he expressed to Jessica as they were leaving the office was . . .

My doctor started me on several medications. Will this be enough to cure me?

THE BOTTOM LINE

It might be a bit disheartening to learn that currently there is no cure for CAD. Once the atherosclerotic plaque has built up in your arteries, it is very difficult to eliminate it. However, the good news is that it *is* possible to control CAD by taking the correct medications and by embracing a healthy lifestyle. It is important to understand that when discussing CAD, the word *control* means "stopping the progression of the disease." By taking medications and changing your lifestyle, you have three goals:

1. Prevent the diagnosed blockage(s) from getting worse.
2. Stop further accumulation of plaque, because this will lead to additional blockages.
3. Prevent possible future heart attacks

Number 2 is especially important, because a diagnosis of one significant blockage (more than 70 percent blocked) is most likely a red flag signaling the potential that other blockages could occur at any time in the future. In fact, this one significant blockage is frequently just a small part of your overall problem. This is because once a critical blockage has been found, it means you have plaque buildup and minor blockages in many, many arteries of your heart (maybe even in other blood vessels of your body). You may not yet have another significant blockage, but without treatment, the accumulation of plaque can quickly move from being 10 or 15 percent to 70 percent or greater blocked, resulting in symptoms or even a heart attack. (Reread Question 4 if you don't remember how this can occur.)

As you may now realize, CAD is a chronic condition that has no cure. However, the good news is that correct and consistent intervention will stall the disease so that it does not progress from minor plaque to a major blockage. Some people are hopeful that a stent or medication cures their heart disease the way antibiotics cure infection. Both medication and a stent can be important, even critical, steps toward improved heart health, but neither is a cure. The stent might fix the one diagnosed critical blockage; however, not all the other arteries of your heart have been fixed. Lifestyle changes and potentially other interventions are necessary, or the plaque will continue to accumulate, resulting in additional critical blockages.

Medication is one of these interventions. In some cases—as with Michael—medication is the initial intervention. If your cardiologist suggests medication as a method for managing your heart disease, keep in mind that medicines always work best in conjunction with a healthy lifestyle. *Medication is **not** a substitution for making healthy choices!* You may want to jump to question 33 for a quick look at how you can begin right now by taking small steps toward becoming healthier, because the most powerful and effective treatment is medication *plus* lifestyle changes. In general, these changes include

1. Quitting smoking.
2. Eating healthily. *(Michael's wife, Dorothy, does the food shopping and cooking. She will have to read chapter 6 to learn what steps to take to help him become healthier.)*
3. Reducing salt intake, especially if you have high blood pressure. *(This is an important change for Michael, since he has high blood pressure that is not very well controlled.)*
4. Getting close to your ideal body weight. *(Michael recognizes that he needs to lose about thirty pounds, and he is ready to take steps to do so.)*
5. Exercising. *(This is where the trouble began for Michael! He began to feel chest pain when he began walking on a treadmill to try to lose weight. Actually, it's a good thing he started exercising, because the red flag chest discomfort allowed the doctor to diagnose his CAD **before** he had a heart attack.)*

In addition to medication and lifestyle management, depending on the results of the stress test, your cardiologist may require further testing, including a coronary angiogram, to determine the extent and severity of your CAD. Your doctor may recommend an angiogram if you have symptoms of CAD (such as chest pain with exertion if you have an abnormal stress test) or if you have significant risk factors for CAD. (In this chapter we will discuss the coronary angiogram in detail.) You should discuss evaluation and treatment options with your cardiologist to determine which evaluative techniques and treatments are best for you. Keep in mind that no matter what other evaluations or treatments your doctor recommends, once you have plaque buildup, it is important to treat it aggressively with medi-cation and lifestyle changes. Even if you receive a stent or endure bypass surgery, you still need to maintain consistent lifestyle changes and take your prescribed medications.

Michael's cardiologist suggested that, in his case, he start with medica-tion and lifestyle changes. She hopes that these will be enough to reduce or eliminate Michael's symptoms. However, she explained to Michael and Dorothy that if Michael's symptoms did not abate after a couple of months, he might need to have further testing.

THE NITTY GRITTY

Medical management of CAD usually consists of a combination of cholesterol medications, blood thinners, and blood pressure medication.

Cholesterol medication

There are different types of cholesterol medications, but those in the class called *statins* are the ones that numerous research studies have shown to be the most beneficial in treating heart disease. The statins received this nickname because the name of each medication in this class or group ends with the suffix -statin. All medications have a pharmaceutical (or scientific) name and a brand name. In this case, statin is the name of the actual pharmaceutical compound. It is not a brand name. The job of statins is to reduce your bad choles-terol (LDL). You can find more about this in Question 28. Statin use has been shown to dramatically decrease the risk of heart attacks, strokes, and death. Unless there is a specific reason not to prescribe a statin, most people with CAD will take one of these cholesterol medications.

Blood thinners

For the majority of people with CAD who have not had angioplasty, a stent, or bypass surgery, you may be surprised to learn that a daily dose of baby aspirin is an effective blood thinner. At low doses, this painkiller decreases the stickiness of platelets in your blood by reducing the platelets' ability to cling to one another. This thins your blood, making it less likely that your blood will form a clot. Some people, however, are allergic to aspirin or may need additional blood thinning. In either of these instances, your doctor may prescribe a blood thinner like Clopidogrel (generic name), otherwise known as Plavix (brand name). You should discuss with your doctor which blood thinner is right for you.

Blood pressure medication

Sometimes a medication for high blood pressure is used to treat CAD. There are different classes of medication used for blood pressure therapy. The class that some studies have found to be beneficial for the treatment of CAD is known as ACE inhibitors. Based upon your history and symptoms, your cardiologist will be able to determine if one of these medications is a good choice for you.

Other medications that may be beneficial in the treatment of CAD include those that treat certain risk factors such as diabetes. The use of these medications is based on an individual's risk factors, and therefore should be determined on a patient-by-patient basis.

It can feel overwhelming to have to take several medications, to think about interventions, and to start to change your lifestyle all at the same time. But don't worry! We will give you the knowledge and tools you need to manage your disease. The steps you will be able to take after reading this book offer you the opportunity to be healthy even though you have been diagnosed with CAD.

QUESTION **13** ————————————

Each day Brian wakes up feeling thankful that he survived his heart attack. His middle child, Matt, graduated from college last month, and Brian knows how fortunate he is to have been able to celebrate with Matt at the graduation ceremony.

Brian has been taking his medication regularly, and one month ago exactly he smoked his last cigarette. He admits that it has been tough to make so many changes, including eating more healthily, but he is doing it because he wants to be around to celebrate many more important milestones with his wife and their three children.

Brian has discovered that, for him, another motivation to staying healthy it is to become as educated as possible about heart disease and the various interventions and treatments that he has had or may have in the future. He frequently thinks back to his time in the emergency room and to the few months after his heart attack, realizing that because everything happened so quickly, there was no time for him to learn the details about the interventions and treatments he had received so far. In addition, in the ER, the medical team also administered a sedating pain medication, which inhibited his memory. Now, Brian wants to understand everything, especially the interventions that saved his life. Specifically, Brian is asking . . .

What is a coronary angiogram?

THE BOTTOM LINE

The prefix *angio-* means "blood vessel," and the suffix -gram means *picture*. You probably know by now that *coronary* refers to the heart. During a coronary angiogram, pictures are taken of the coronary blood vessels, or arteries.

Brian was interested to learn that an angiogram can actually be conducted on many other blood vessels in the body. For example, a cerebral angiogram means that images are taken of the blood vessels in the brain.

An angiogram is an *invasive procedure*. The definition of an invasive procedure is that something is inserted into your body for the duration of the procedure. An angiogram is *not* considered surgery, because no cutting is involved. In the case of a coronary angiogram, a catheter, or small tube, is inserted into a blood vessel and then moved all the way into your coronary artery.

Since an angiogram takes pictures (images) of the arterial system (specifically the coronary artery), your doctor requires access to your arterial system through a major artery. Typically, access is obtained via your arm (through an artery in your wrist) or, much more routinely, via your leg, through the artery in your groin (Figure 5). By *access*, we mean that a blood vessel in your wrist or groin is punctured with a small needle, and then a small tube (called an *access sheath*) is placed into the artery (similar to having an IV placed). Once the sheath has been placed, the needle is removed. The procedure is most often conducted through the artery in the groin because it is technically more challenging to go through the arm (see more about this in The Nitty Gritty).

Once the doctor has the access sheath (known as a *work tube*) in place, to access a main artery, another small, hollow tube (called

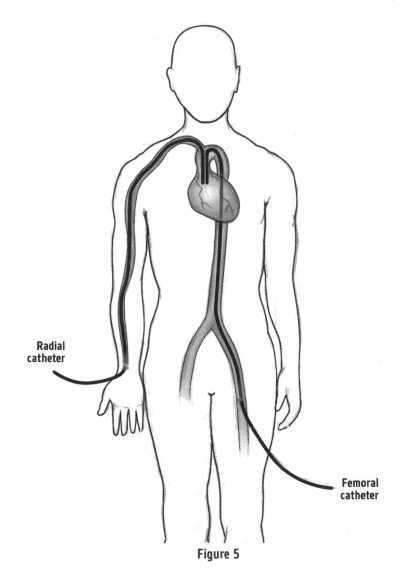

**Radial
catheter**

**Femoral
catheter**

Figure 5

a *catheter*) is placed inside the first tube and advanced through the arteries in your body, all the way to the heart. Pretty amazing, right! The first, short tube remains stationary, keeping the puncture site open for the catheter. The catheter has a shaped tip, which permits easy maneuvering and traveling through the arteries (Figure 5). Your doctor may try a few different catheters until one is found that fits your specific anatomy. This is easily accomplished with access through the first tube, which doesn't move until the angiogram has been completed.

Once the catheter has reached the coronary artery, the next step of the procedure takes place. The catheter itself is not inserted all the way through the coronary arteries. Rather, once the catheter reaches the beginning of the correct blood vessel, the cardiologist will begin to inject a contrast dye into your heart's arteries (Figure 6). This is important, because blood can't be seen on an x-ray but dye can be. The contrast dye fills the entire coronary artery system, and while the dye is in the coronary arteries, x-ray images are taken of the blood vessels. These images can be seen on a monitor.

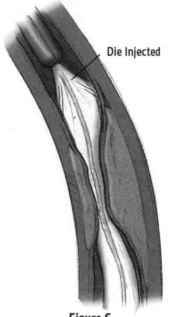

Die Injected

Figure 6

Brian vaguely remembers this part—the big machine hanging above his body as he lay on the table. He recalls it moving at times, but he can't remember why . . .

The camera is about the size of a toaster oven, and it is suspended above the table on which you will be lying throughout the procedure.

Each time dye is inserted through the catheter, the camera is rotated in order to obtain video loops of the blood vessels from different angles. The camera may move closer to your head at times, and depending on the camera's angle, you may be asked to move your head or to take a deep breath. You will be awake yet relaxed and comfortable during the procedure, so you will be able to follow this type of simple direction. By taking pictures from all different angles, your doctor will be better able to identify blockages, and then determine the exact location of any blockages. The images are actually small videos, recording five or ten seconds at a time. On a monitor, the cardiologist is able to see your beating heart and watch the dye flowing through the coronary arteries. If there are blockages or plaque buildups, the dye will highlight this as a narrowing in the blood vessels. X-rays are taken from *outside* your body, by a camera situated above your chest.

As part of this procedure, your doctor may decide to take a picture of the main heart chamber in addition to the coronary arteries. This allows your doctor to evaluate your heart function much like an echocardiogram (see Question 9). This evaluation is separate from the coronary angiogram but conducted at the same time.

If your doctor decides to take this step, a catheter is advanced into the main chamber of the heart (the left ventricle), and then dye is injected directly into the ventricle. You might feel a few heart palpitations (skipped heartbeats) during this part of the procedure, but this will only last a couple of seconds and is not at all dangerous. As the dye is injected into your heart, you will experience a warm feeling spreading throughout your body. Your doctor may even warn you when to expect this sensation. This, too, is completely normal and will remit in less than a minute.

The entire procedure should take no longer than about half an hour. Keep in mind that this is only a *diagnostic* procedure. Nothing is fixed during the coronary angiogram! However, if, during this evaluation, your doctor determines that angioplasty is needed (as was the case with Brian when he had his heart attack), this second procedure is typically done immediately, directly after the angiogram. The angioplasty will add additional time to the procedure. If you want to learn more about angioplasty, you can jump directly to Question 18.

Once the angiogram (and angioplasty, if needed) has been completed, the catheter is removed through the access tube, and then the access tube must also be removed from the artery. The removal of the access tube will vary depending upon which site is used. If a wrist artery is used, the tube is simply removed, and a band is placed around the wrist to compress the artery, which prevents bleeding. If a groin artery is used, once the tube is removed, pressure must be applied to prevent bleeding. Usually, this is accomplished by a nurse or aid compressing the spot by hand. This manual compression lasts for fifteen minutes to ensure that the bleeding has stopped. Admittedly, this compression might feel uncomfortable or even painful. If it feels very painful, don't hesitate to ask for pain medication. As an alternative, some facilities have devices that close the hole at the end of the procedure, when the tube is removed. This eliminates the need to apply pressure. You might ask your doctor if you are a candidate for this.

After the procedure, you will be moved to a recovery area, where you will be closely monitored for a few hours. If your procedure was conducted through the groin area, you will need to lie still for a few hours so the puncture site can heal. If a wrist artery was used, you will be able to sit up, but you will have only limited use of that arm, as long as the band is still on your wrist. Under most circumstances, you may eat and drink while you recover from the procedure.

THE NITTY GRITTY

Your cardiologist should make the ultimate decision as to which artery should be used to insert the tube for this procedure. If you have a preference, you should certainly discuss this with your doctor.

In most instances, your doctor will elect to use the right side of your groin or arm as the access site, since this is the side of the table on which the doctor stands. However, there are times that it is preferable to choose the left side; for example, if you have a blockage in your right leg or if you have had multiple procedures in the area, resulting in significant scar tissue. In this case the doctor will have to lean slightly over you to access the left side. But don't worry!

Brian remembered that his angiogram had been done through his groin. He couldn't help thinking that his wrist seemed so much more convenient, so he's wondering whether there is a good reason to choose the groin . . .

The main advantage to access the artery through the wrist is that there is slightly less risk of bleeding and less pain during removal of the tube. (See Questions 20–22 for more discussions about potential complications of this procedure.) In addition, you have greater mobility during recovery (since you don't have to lie flat on your back until the bleeding has stopped).

On the other hand, it is technically more challenging to use the wrist for access, so fewer doctors offer this procedure. Also, accessing through the wrist might be a bit more painful because this blood vessel is smaller than the one in the groin. What's more, since the groin blood vessel is larger, it will accommodate slightly larger tubes and catheters, giving your doctor more equipment options from which to choose. You can discuss all these considerations with your interventional cardiologist, but ultimately let him or her assess your medical condition and decide which option is best for you.

Myth 1

Contrary to popular belief, the camera taking video images of your arteries is *not* attached to the catheter or placed inside your body in any way. As described above, the catheter is used only to inject dye into the coronary arteries and the camera is outside the body. This misconception is understandable, because there are other procedures—like colonoscopies or other gastrointestinal procedures—in which a camera is actually placed inside your body. This is not possible for an angiogram because the space used (a blood vessel) is a tiny fraction of the size of your intestine, so there is no space for a camera.

Myth 2

Another misconception is that groin access for the catheter is via a man's penis or a woman's urethra or vagina. In fact, the catheter used to capture urine during some procedures (a bladder or Foley catheter) has nothing in common with the catheters used for coronary angiogram. During an angiogram, the blood vessel is accessed in the area above your hip, not through your genitals.

Brian benefited from learning the details about the angiogram. To begin, he was glad to know more about the procedure that had helped to save his life. Having knowledge also helped him realize that should he ever need another angiogram he will be emotionally equipped to handle the procedure, now that he has a full understanding about what to expect.

QUESTION 14

Reginald's stress test results indicated that he is at high risk for CAD, and his doctor said that he definitely requires an angiogram. Reginald is very nervous about having the procedure. In addition, if he is honest with himself, he doesn't feel like he has a great support system. His wife, Ida, seems more annoyed than worried about his stress test result. She blames his weight gain for his problems.

"I've been telling him for years to do something about his weight and to stop smoking," complained Ida. "I guess high blood pressure isn't enough. Maybe he needs to have a heart attack to be able to see the writing on the wall!"

Since he doesn't want to upset Ida any more than she is already, Reginald hasn't been sharing his feelings with anyone, not even his doctors, his buddy Marcus, or the guys down at the senior center. Of course, this has been increasing his stress level even more. If Reginald was able to confront his feelings, he might ask . . .

I don't want to admit it, but I'm nervous about getting an angiogram. What does it feel like?

THE BOTTOM LINE

Reginald would be comforted to know that, while almost no medical procedure is comfortable, there is typically no significant pain associated with a coronary angiogram. The primary reason that people may be anxious about the procedure is a worry associated with knowing that a catheter will be moving through their body and especially around or into their heart.

It is certainly understandable that you may be worried. It is important, however, to remember that this procedure is performed with no problems on millions of people worldwide. Generally, it is a very safe procedure with a low rate of complications. Prior to the procedure, most patients receive a mild sedative, such as Valium or Benadryl. This helps to calm you if you feel very anxious.

I feel a bit better with that information. What should I expect?

To begin, you will be required to not eat or drink for at least six to eight hours prior to the procedure. The exact number of hours for fasting will vary, depending upon your doctor or hospital. Therefore, prior to the procedure, be sure to ask for instructions as to how long you should fast.

Reginald's doctor asked him to fast for eight hours. Since his procedure was in the early morning, Reginald didn't find the fasting too challenging, because he was asleep most of the time.

On the day of your procedure, you will begin in a pre-procedure area where you will be prepped before you enter the catheterization laboratory (the room in which you will have your procedure). At this time, several steps will be taken:

1. You will receive an IV that will remain connected to you throughout the procedure. This allows the medical team to administer intravenous medication during the procedure (see The Nitty Gritty for more information about this).
2. You will receive IV fluids before, during, and for a short while after the procedure. This ensures that you stay hydrated, and it also flushes the x-ray dye out of your system.
3. If access to your arteries will be through the groin area (see Question 13), this area might be shaved so that it is free of hair and easy to clean.
4. Several EKG stickers, necessary to attach EKG leads, will be stuck onto your chest. If your chest is very hairy, some areas may be shaved in order to ensure that the stickers will properly adhere.

Once the prep is completed, you will be moved to the procedure room (the catheterization laboratory, or cath lab). The cath lab looks very similar to a surgical room but for the fact that it contains large x-ray equipment. At this time, you will be placed onto the x-ray table. This is a somewhat narrow, hard table constructed to allow x-rays to pass through it. Admittedly, it is not a comfortable surface, but most people have no problem with it for the short duration of the procedure. If you have back pain, however, or any other problem that makes this table extremely uncomfortable for you, make sure to request IV pain medication.

Reginald did not have a problem lying on the table for the procedure.

Once you are situated on the table, your arms will be strapped onto arm boards. These will ensure that you stay in place during the angiogram, although you need to remember not to move too much during the procedure. Next, your entire body (except your head) will be covered with a sterile cover. It is very important not to touch this cover after it has been placed on you, because doing so would compromise the sterile field and expose you to the risk of infection. Therefore, when you get an inevitable nose itch, be sure to keep your arms in the arm boards. Don't be embarrassed to ask a nurse to scratch your nose; your medical team is there to help you! The sterile cover will have a hole in the region through which the procedure will be performed. If this is your groin, your genitals will be covered at all times.

A few minutes after being covered, Reginald felt like he had something irritating the inside of his eye. He told the nurse, and she gently wiped his eye with a piece of gauze. It worked, and Reginald felt comfortable for the rest of the procedure.

At this point, due to the IV sedation and pain medication that you have been receiving, you should feel very calm. Ideally, you should be relaxed, slightly drowsy, but awake rather than completely asleep, as you would be for major surgery. This is called *conscious sedation*.

There are several advantages to your being awake during an angiogram procedure (in addition to the fact that it is not supposed to be a painful procedure). Most important, receiving general anesthetic holds some risks, especially for individuals with heart disease. In addition, receiving sedation rather than general anesthesia means that your recovery from the procedure will be quicker. It is also helpful for your doctor to be able to communicate with you during the procedure. This is because you may need to follow a few simple directions such as turning your head or holding your breath. Since you are conscious, if you feel any unusual discomfort, you will be able to tell your doctor, and he or she will immediately adjust the catheter or give you more pain medication.

Once the doctor is satisfied that you have received adequate medication, the access site (wrist or groin) will be cleaned with iodine (a cold liquid that sterilizes the area). This may feel slightly uncomfortable, but it should be only for a few seconds.

When you have been fully prepared for the procedure, your doctor will feel for the pulse in your wrist or groin to determine the position at which access will be found. Next, the doctor will apply a local anesthetic (like the type you get in a dentist's office), which will numb the area. This may burn for about thirty seconds, until the anesthetic begins to work. Most people feel a slight discomfort when the tube is inserted into the artery, but this typically lasts less than a minute or so. In fact, once the tube is in place, you can relax and not worry about any discomfort or pain. This is because there are no nerves on the inside of blood vessels, so you will not feel the catheter moving through your arteries.

Reginald's doctor elected to use the right groin for access. Reginald was surprised that, despite his worrying, he felt very little discomfort as the procedure began.

There is not much for you to do, except perhaps move your head one way or another, should your doctor determine that it is in the way of a particular camera angle. You might also occasionally be asked to take a deep breath or to hold your breath. Throughout the procedure, you will notice that the lights turn off at times. The lights are part of the x-ray machine, and they automatically turn off when the doctor uses the x-ray machine to capture and view video of your arteries and heart. The reason for this is analogous to having the lights turned off in a movie theater, that is, it is easier to see the screen in a darkened room.

Suddenly the doctor was telling Reginald that the procedure was over. He breathed a sigh of relief and realized that it had been much quicker than he had expected and not at all painful.

THE NITTY GRITTY

In most cases, it is quite simple for your cardiologist to access your artery to begin the angiogram. However, if you have had this procedure multiple times in the past, it can be a bit more difficult to get to the artery. This is because scar tissue can form around the blood vessel, which makes it difficult to locate the vessel and then access it with the needle and tube. In this case, it is possible that the beginning of procedure will be a little more painful. If you are in this situation, you might discuss with your doctor the possibility of using a different access site. For example, if your right groin area has been accessed many times in the past—and therefore is more sensitive— ask the doctor to use your left groin area. Also, don't hesitate to ask your doctor for additional sedation and more local anesthetic.

Conscious sedation does an excellent job of ensuring that the angiogram is as stress-free as possible. In fact, you may even fall asleep briefly during the procedure. This is normal, and you shouldn't fight it. If it is necessary for you to be alert at any point, the doctor or nurse will awaken you.

Under very special circumstances, such as if a patient has an extreme phobia, the procedure can be accomplished using general anesthesia. This is not ideal, and it poses a greater risk. Nevertheless, for some people, it may be better to have general anesthesia than to have a panic attack during the procedure. If you believe that you may need general anesthesia, talk to your doctor well *in advance* of the procedure, because scheduling general anesthesia cannot be done at the last minute. Of course, ultimately it is your doctor who must decide whether, medically, general anesthesia is in your best interest.

In addition to painkillers and sedatives, sometimes other medications are administered through the catheter directly into the coronary arteries. Nitroglycerin, the most commonly used medication, helps dilate (enlarge) the blood vessels to prevent them from going into spasm. Some people experience headaches when they are given nitroglycerin, but this should resolve within ten to fifteen minutes, unless multiple doses are used.

QUESTION **15** ─────────

When Rosa first arrived at the ER, the doctors quickly diagnosed her heart attack and rushed her into the cath lab for a coronary angiogram, followed immediately (during the same procedure, utilizing the same catheter) by an angioplasty (stent placement).

After the catheter was removed from her groin, a nurse applied pressure to the area for about fifteen to twenty minutes to prevent bleeding. Then, in the cardiac intensive care unit (CCU), Rosa began her recovery from the heart attack and the angiogram–angioplasty. After the removal of the catheter, Rosa was told to lie flat for another four to six hours. She was monitored in the CCU for a couple of days, and then she was moved to a regular room. Since she was recovering well, she was released from the hospital at the end of the third day. During her hospital stay, a nurse carefully monitored Rosa to make sure she had no bleeding in her groin, the area in which the catheter had been placed.

But my situation is different to Rosa's.
My doctor did not say that I would have to stay in the hospital overnight.

As you may realize, in many cases, an angiogram is not conducted in an emergency situation (the result of a heart attack). It is often an elective procedure, which means it is planned because someone is exhibiting concerning symptoms. If this is the reason that you are having an angiogram, you may not require an overnight stay at the hospital. If you only have the diagnostic angiogram, you will be discharged once you have sufficiently recovered. Since you will usually need to recover for at least four to six hours, you will still spend a full day at a hospital. Just as the nurse kept an eye on Rosa for three days, to make sure that she didn't begin bleeding, you will need to do this for yourself. (Don't worry. Later we will talk more about how to monitor yourself.) However, if you also receive a stent, you will likely be required to stay overnight.

When Rosa was released from the hospital, she wanted to make sure that she continued to recover well so she could be back to her usual routine as soon as possible. Rosa's most pressing question is . . .

Now that the procedure is over and I'm recovering, are there any precautions I should take?

THE BOTTOM LINE

It is important to know that complications following an angiogram are uncommon and generally avoidable by carefully following your doctor's recommendations. Just as preparations *before* a coronary angiogram or angioplasty may vary slightly between hospitals or doctors, so too might recommendations *after* discharge from the hospital. In addition, every patient is different, so it is important to follow *your* doctor's recommendations carefully rather than take the advice of a friend or family member who may have had the procedure.

On the rare occasion that you experience a complication after an angiogram, it is typically in one of two places:

1. In the area of your heart
2. In the area surrounding the access area

Your heart

If your heart or heart vessels are injured during the procedure, you might experience complications. However, please remember that it is extremely rare to have problems like this. The signs that your heart might have been injured during an angiogram are the same as those when you are having a heart attack. Therefore, at any point after you have been released from the hospital, if you experience chest tightness, pressure, or other signs (see Question 1), you must *seek medical attention right away*, especially if the pain does not resolve. If the heart or a heart vessel is injured, the doctor can usually repair the damage as soon as the symptoms appear. It is therefore important for you to be as vigilant as possible for possible symptoms associated with a heart attack.

Rosa had no signs of discomfort or pain in the area of her heart in the days following the procedure. Since she had already been through a lot, she was happy that this went well.

The access site

Although it is not common, it is possible to develop bleeding in the area that was the access site for the catheter. Bleeding from an access site does not necessarily mean the blood will be visible or that it will actually leak out from your body (like when you cut yourself). In fact, most of the time you will *not* see any blood. Rather, if there is leakage from an artery, you will feel blood accumulating under your skin, and the area will start to feel swollen. This accumulation could grow to the size of a golf ball or even a tennis ball. This type of swelling, known as a *hematoma*, will feel rubbery and firm, and it is usually very painful, so it is not easily missed.

Although bleeding is rare, it occurs more commonly when the groin is used as the access site. Therefore, if your angiogram was through your groin, it is important to check on the site each day for signs of swelling. You should continue to check for about a week after the procedure. The most effective way to check is by applying slight pressure with your hand in the groin area. It is a good idea to try this technique before you leave the hospital so that you know how it feels when there is no swelling (it shouldn't feel very different from the side that was not used during the procedure.)

Whether the procedure was through your groin or your wrist, don't worry if you see a black and blue mark (bruise) in the area, because this is very common. It does indicate a very small amount of bleeding under the skin, but it is nothing to be concerned about, even if it is quite large. This is different from a hematoma, which will feel swollen and firm. Of course, if you are unsure whether what you are seeing or feeling is a hematoma, it is always best to ask your doctor.

If the procedure was through your wrist, you should pay attention to whether there is any bleeding or swelling around the wrist and throughout the arm, all the way up to your armpit. In the very rare circumstance that you develop unusual pain in your arm, become unable to move your hand, or if you lose sensation in your hand or fingers, *you must see a doctor immediately*. But don't be too concerned about these potential complications, because they are *very* unlikely to occur.

When Rosa took a look at her body a couple of hours after the procedure, she discovered that she had a huge bruise in her right groin. At first she was upset, but then she remembered that this was normal and nothing to worry about. Except for a little tenderness at the site for a day or two, this was the only side effect she had from the procedure.

What can I do to prevent bleeding?

Following your doctor's directions when you are discharged is the very best way to make sure the access site doesn't bleed. If your procedure was done through the groin, the most important recommendation you will receive is to avoid activities that put a lot of pressure on the groin. Many doctors will advise you not to drive for a couple of days, not to exercise (running, biking, etc.) for about a week, and not to lift anything over twenty pounds for a week or two. If you lift an object that is too heavy, you might feel a *pop*, which means that the seal at the access site has been dislodged. This is not a sensation you want to have, so don't overexert yourself. It is usually fine to lie down, sit up, walk, and use the stairs. However, local standards vary, and you must ask your doctor for specific instructions in case your procedure was more complicated than usual.

If the procedure was through the artery in your wrist, you will be asked to avoid activities that require excessive use of this arm and wrist. In addition, you should avoid driving for a couple of days, and you should rest the arm as much as possible. You should also avoid lifting heavy objects, including your suitcase when you leave the hospital. You have a good excuse to avoid household chores for a couple of days!

Rosa found it especially difficult to have to give up baby-sitting her grandchildren for a while. She missed them, and she felt bad because she knew that it was difficult for her daughter, Lisa, to juggle work and the kids each day after school. Nevertheless, Rosa realized that the best way to get back to her grandkids quickly was to take the necessary time to heal from the heart attack and procedure. Lisa assured her that they would manage, and that she should come back to baby-sitting when she was ready. During her recovery, Lisa brought Chloe and Nick to visit Rosa, and before long she was beginning to feel better.

Is that all I should know about?

Another very uncommon complication is infection at the access site. Signs of infection include redness around the site, localized swelling (not a hematoma), and sometimes pus (a yellow or green discharge) from the access site. When an infection is more advanced, you might experience a fever and a general feeling of malaise. However, remember, infection is very rare and unlikely to be dangerous if you see your doctor immediately. Therefore, don't worry too much now that you know how to recognize the symptoms.

To reduce the chance of infection, until the scab falls of the wound, you should avoid swimming or bathing in a tub. There is potentially a lot of bacteria in swimming pool and tub water that could come into contact with your healing wound. It is fine to shower, as long as you avoid excessive scrubbing or manipulation of the access site.

There are no specific dietary restrictions after having an angio-gram–angioplasty. However, remember that a heart healthy diet is absolutely key for your future well-being (see more on healthy diets in chapter 6).

Rosa decided that she wants to live a long time—to share life with her kids and grandkids. She has already begun thinking about what changes she needs to make in order to prevent another heart attack.

THE NITTY GRITTY

The catheter is inserted without the need for cutting (as would be necessary for a surgical procedure). Therefore, you will not require stitches that must be removed. Instead, there is a small puncture wound that usually develops a scab quite quickly. This wound will be covered with a small bandage when you leave the hospital. It is best to leave the bandage on for a couple of days or until it falls off. The scab will naturally fall off by itself, and the wound should be completely healed within a week or two. Since this procedure requires no cutting of the skin, once the wound has healed, there should be no scarring.

Recovery from an angiogram is quite easy with very little risk for complications. However, if you experience any concerning symptoms, contact your doctor or go to the emergency room. Other important symptoms that require immediate attention include stomach or back pain, feeling weak, low blood pressure, or difficulty breathing.

QUESTION **16**

Diane worried about having a coronary angiogram, particularly because her chronic back pain makes it difficult for her to lie still for a long time (especially on a hard table). However, having the procedure through her wrist really made a difference, because she was able to sit up immediately after the procedure. If the doctor had used groin access, she would have had to rest on her back for four to six hours after the procedure. The doctor also made sure that Diane received sufficient pain and sedative medication throughout the procedure so that she didn't feel a lot of back pain. As a result, Diane was relatively comfortable and only remembers a little of the procedure.

Once Diane woke up from the procedure, her cardiologist reviewed the results of the angiogram. The news wasn't great, though. Her doctor reported that the angiogram showed many blockages in Diane's coronary arteries.

Diane tried to focus on everything the doctor was saying to her, but the most pressing question that kept going through her mind was . . .

My angiogram showed that I have a blockage in my heart artery. What are my options now?

THE BOTTOM LINE

Once a coronary angiogram identifies one or more blockages, three possible options will be considered in order to minimize any further damage to the heart or arteries. These three treatment options include

1. **Treatment with medication but no other intervention.** Monitor to make sure that your symptoms don't worsen.
2. **Open the blockage with angioplasty.** This usually means that a stent has been placed.
3. **Perform bypass surgery.**

For the most part, you will rely on your cardiologist to recommend which treatment option is right for you. There are several factors that will impact her recommendation. Of these, the three most important factors are

1. **The anatomy of your coronary arteries.** Your doctor will assess how many blockages you have and precisely where these blockages are. This is important because some blockages are better treated with stents and some with bypass.

Diane's angiogram revealed that she has many blockages, possibly too many to treat with stents.

2. **Your risk factors.** There are several risk factors to consider: how well your heart muscle is functioning (the ejection fraction; see Question 9 for), whether you have diabetes or other diseases, and your age (some very elderly patients may not be good candidates for surgery).

Diane has diabetes, but her ejection fraction (heart function) is normal. This is great, because it means that there is no damage to the heart muscle itself.

3. **Your symptoms.** The type and severity of your symptoms will help determine the best treatment option. For example, your doctor will assess whether you have chest pain with exertion as well as how frequently this happens and how long the pain lasts.

Diane does not have any symptoms, but this may be misleading in her case because she is very sedentary due to the arthritis in her back.

As you can see, your doctor's recommendation will be based upon many sometimes complex factors. Your treatment will be tailored to meet your needs. It is therefore important to resist the urge to compare yourself to anyone else you know who has seen a cardiologist for similar concerns. Your doctor will carefully take into account all clinical factors and make an educated recommendation. In general, if you have many symptoms, your doctor is less likely to recommend medication alone. However, if you have only one blockage in a smaller branch vessel and little symptoms, it might be sufficient to treat with medication and monitor your situation carefully.

You do not need to worry about making any medical decisions, because your cardiologist will consider all your medical issues before making a recommendation. However, it is important to discuss all your options with your doctor and ask her to explain the reasons for her recommendation. It is important for you to understand this clearly. If, for any reason, you aren't sure that you are comfortable with your cardiologist's recommendation, you can always get a second opinion. Remember, this is your body and your health, which means that it is your *right* to feel completely comfortable with the medical decisions affecting your life. In fact, most doctors are supportive of their patients seeking more than one opinion before making a major medical decision.

Will fixing the blockages with stents or even bypass surgery save my life?

This is a great question asked by many people—even cardiologists! The answer is not as simple as you might think, though. If you are actually having a heart attack, a stent or bypass can *definitely* save your life! It is therefore *extremely important* for you to call 911 without delay if you or someone near you appears to be having a heart attack.

The answer, however, is not as simple if you are having chest pain with exertion, or like Diane, you have blockages and multiple risk factors without chest pain. Most people who have had a stent procedure, or even those who understand a little about angioplasty, believe that opening a blockage will prevent a future heart attack and thereby save a life. Interestingly, however, some research indicates that stents do not prevent future heart attacks or lengthen the life span of people who have only mild symptoms. Although stents *are* effective in reducing or eliminating chest pain, they may not help you live longer or stop you from having another heart attack. This is understandable when you remember that the discovery of a first blockage is often a warning symptom. The stent addresses only the blockage that has been discovered; it does not treat any others that might exist.

There is a great deal of continuing research in the scientific community to continue learning who will most benefit from a stent or a bypass and who should begin with medication alone. At this time, research tells us that patients at highest risk benefit most from receiving a stent and should therefore have the procedure. Patients at lower risk can usually try medication first, if they are reluctant to have the procedure. After trying the medication for a while, you will be able to tell if it is helping your chest pain. In some cases you will still require a future stent for this blockage or for another one.

THE NITTY GRITTY

It bears repeating that there is *clear scientific evidence* from numerous studies that if you are having a heart attack, you will do *much* better if you seek emergency medical attention *immediately*. The sooner a blockage can be opened with a stent, the greater your chances for reduced damage to your heart muscle and the lower your risk of death. *Under no circumstances should you delay calling 911 if you think you may be having a heart attack.*

The debate about whether a stent will save a life focuses on stable patients. This means that you have some degree of coronary artery blockage that causes occasional chest pain with exertion. There are no signs of a heart attack (see more about angina in Question 4).

Two recent studies addressed this debate.[8] In both studies, patients were randomly assigned to one of two treatment groups (they were assigned by chance, with a fifty-fifty chance that a patient would get into either group). Randomization in research is important so that particular patient traits or factors are distributed evenly between two groups that are being studied. For the initial treatment of blockages, the first group of patients was given only medication, and the second group was given medication plus a stent. Then these patients were followed by the researchers for several years. During the follow-up period, about one-third of the patients in the medication-only group subsequently required a stent procedure. In addition, the medication-plus-stent group experienced greater relief from chest pain. Based on this and numerous other studies, it is clear that a stent procedure is a very effective way to treat chest pain, allowing an individual to return to regular activities and lifestyle.

However, the study did not reveal a reduction in heart attacks or death when stents were used as compared to the patients treated with medication alone. At the time this finding was released, it led to some articles in the nonscientific press (newspapers, magazines, etc.) that asserted stents are overused and unnecessary. Unfortunately, many of these articles were either very one-sided or they did not recognize the limitations of the research (or both). In fact, many leading cardiologists have criticized these two studies for a variety of shortcomings.

The debate continues among cardiologists worldwide as to the best treatment options for patients in the stable angina group. There are currently two studies under way that will attempt to clarify which patients benefit most from treating blockages with medication alone and which require a stent or bypass.

Until further research has been completed, we rely on the current research and experience. For now, it is clear that patients who have had a heart attack or who have unstable symptoms will benefit from stents. This group of patients will see a reduction in deaths and recurrent heart attacks. The group of patients with stable symptoms will have improvement in their symptoms, but it is unclear if they will have better outcomes with respect to death and heart attack.

CHAPTER

Four

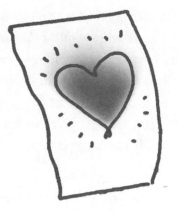

Which Treatment Is Right for Me?

QUESTION **17** ———————

While lying in the recovery area, Reginald is nervous because he is waiting for the doctor to tell him the results of the angiogram. Before the procedure, he had told himself that, whatever the results, he would deal with it. But now that he is about to learn whether he will need further treatment, Reginald worries that it could be bad news. Eventually, after what seems like an eternity (but was really only twenty minutes), his cardiologist arrives at his bedside and offers his diagnosis and recommended treatment plan. Reginald, though prepared for the worst, is surprised to hear that while his heart does have several blockages, none is severe enough to require a stent or bypass surgery. Instead, the doctor feels that the best treatment is medication and a change of lifestyle. Reginald thinks about the chest pain he has been having and immediately wonders . . .

Is medication alone enough to make me feel better?

THE BOTTOM LINE

The results of a cardiac angiogram fall into one of three general categories:

1. **Severe blockage** (about 70 percent or more blocked): Significantly impairs blood flow to the heart. The blockages can be repaired with either one or more stents or with bypass surgery.
2. **Intermediate blockage** (about 50 to 70 percent blocked): May or may not impair blood flow to the heart. Further testing is required to determine if stent or bypass surgery is necessary.

3. **No blockage or minor blockage** (less than 50 percent): Does not impair blood flow to the heart. Requires only medication and lifestyle changes to treat successfully.

Reginald's angiogram revealed that he fell into category 2. His doctor found several blockages of intermediate significance as determined by the angiogram.

However, an angiogram doesn't tell the whole story. An angiogram reveals the *anatomic* information about a blockage—meaning the percentage of blockage—but even that is somewhat subjective, as a 50 percent blockage may be 40 percent to one doctor and 60 percent to another. In addition, the angiographic appearance of a blockage does not always tell us the *hemodynamic significance* of the blockage. This is a fancy way of saying that the angiogram may not be able to determine whether the blockage actually impairs blood flow to the heart (*hemo* means "blood," and *dynamic* means "movement").

His doctor explained to Reginald that when a blockage is less than 50 percent, it almost never obstructs blood flow and therefore does not require a stent.

On the other hand, a blockage of more than 80 percent almost always impairs blood flow. Finally, when a blockage falls in the 50–70 percent range (like Reginald's blockages), blood flow to the heart is only sometimes impaired and therefore doesn't always require a stent. Reginald was surprised to learn that a blockage of more than 50 percent might not impair blood flow, but his doctor explained that until the blockage is around 70 percent, the body is often able to compensate so that blood flow to the heart muscle does not decrease. When a blockage falls into this middle range, it is important to conduct further testing to determine whether the heart muscle is, in fact, receiving less blood than it should.

A stress test (as described earlier) is one way of evaluating the hemodynamic significance of a blockage. However, as we have discussed, stress tests are not always 100 percent accurate. A more accurate method of assessing blockages is a test called FFR (*fractional flow reserve*, see details about this test in The Nitty Gritty).

When Reginald's doctor conducted an FFR on his blockages, the test revealed that his blockages did not impair the blood flow to his heart enough to require a stent. Reginald's doctor, therefore, recommended that the only treatment he requires at this time is medication and a healthier lifestyle.

Wouldn't it be better to just fix it anyway to prevent the blockage from getting worse or just in case . . .

This is a good question because it seems logical to just open up the clog the way you would a drain, except the human body is *not* a drain. Angioplasty is a very safe procedure, but it is not completely risk free. Consider this along with the fact that there is no benefit to placing a stent in a blockage that does not impair blood flow. In this case, one would have the risk of the procedure without the potential benefit. In fact, there have been studies that evaluated this issue. Their results revealed that patients who received stents in blockages that did not impair blood flow actually had less satisfactory outcomes than patients treated with only medication.[9, 10] Even more important, patients who have intermediate blockages that do not impair blood flow to the heart and receive *only* medication have a very good prognosis (chance for improved health) for many years after the initial coronary angiogram.[11] Based on these studies, most interventional cardiologists believe that, in the majority of cases, angioplasty is not recommended when blockages do not impair blood flow (including blockages below about 70 percent).

That seems quite easy. All I need to do is take a pill and I'll be okay?

Not exactly. The best treatment for nonsignificant blockages is called *optimal medical therapy*, which is a combination of medication and lifestyle changes. To be optimally treated does not just mean taking medications; it means reaching specific goals for cholesterol, blood pressure, and blood sugar levels (see chapter 6). In order to reach these goals, medication is very helpful, but living more healthily and kicking bad habits (like smoking) are also *very* important. For Reginald this means he must stay away from cigarettes.

When Reginald learned that his doctor recommended against angio-plasty for his blockages, he was not actually happy. Reginald had hoped for a quick fix, which would let him get back to living his life in the way he had been living it, which for the most part he enjoyed (except for the money stresses and the fights with Ida). Reginald's cardiologist disagreed, however.

"You are very fortunate that the blockages were discovered before they caused a heart attack or had a chance to impair the blood flow to your heart." What's more, explained the doctor, "If you take your medi-cation as prescribed and do your part to becoming healthier, there is an excellent chance that these blockages will not cause you any problems for a long time to come."

Reginald felt a little better after the doctor reassured him that he would still be able to lead a healthy, active life. Reginald's first step toward better health was to talk to his wife.

"Ida, go home and throw out all the cigarettes in the house. I don't want to be tempted to smoke even one of them." Ida nodded in agreement.

"Reginald," she said, "the next thing we need to do is work on fight-ing less often. That will reduce your stress, which will make you less likely to want to smoke!"

Reginald smiled at Ida. Maybe something good would come of this scare after all!

THE NITTY GRITTY

As you now know, an angiogram alone is sometimes not sufficient to determine how bad a blockage is. This is because there are many factors in addition to the degree of blockage that can influence how much the blockage actually reduces blood flow to the heart. Some of these factors have to do with the blockage itself (the degree and length of the blockage or if there are multiple blockages). Other factors relate to the part of the heart muscle that receives blood from the blocked artery how much heart muscle is supplied by the blocked blood vessel and if the person has had a prior heart attack).

Sometimes, if the heart muscle has been damaged by a prior heart attack, the heart may not require full blood flow. For instance, this works much in the same way as watering a lawn. If the entire lawn is green (a healthy heart), it will require the full amount of water necessary to keep it hydrated and alive (full blood flow). However, if part of the lawn is already brown and lifeless (a heart with permanent damage caused by a prior heart attack), it doesn't require the full amount of water to keep it alive, and in fact, less water may be providing more than adequate water (limited blood flow may be enough, even if there is a blockage).

The test we mentioned above, the FFR (*fractional flow reserve*), is used to determine if a blockage is impairing blood flow in a detrimental way to the heart (*hemodynamic significance*). The FFR test is quite simple: it measures the pressure in the artery before and after the blockage (Figure 7). A small wire is inserted into the coronary artery downstream of the blockage (after the blockage). A tiny pressure transducer on this wire measures the pressure inside the coronary artery. Then the pressure after the blockage is compared to the pressure before the blockage. If there is no significant impairment of blood flow, there should be no drop (or only a minimal drop) in blood pressure when comparing the pressure before and after the blocked area. However, if there *is* a significant blockage, the pressure beyond the blockage drops substantially, indicating that the

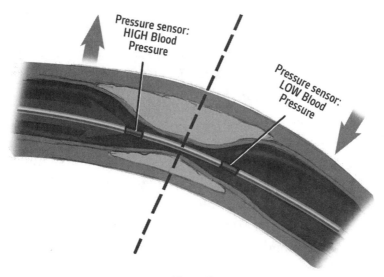

Figure 7

blood flow to the heart is impaired. In such instances, the blockage is considered significant, and most cardiologists will recommend treatment with angioplasty (a stent) or bypass surgery.

To conduct this test, it is necessary to simulate a stress test that allows a cardiologist to see the vessel while blood is pumping through it vigorously. To accomplish this, a medication is given to the patient via IV that causes the heart to pump blood as if the patient were exercising (this is very similar to the chemical stress test described in Question 8). The cardiologist is able to check each blockage separately to determine which may be causing a problem. During the infusion of the medication, you may experience some chest discomfort, burning in your chest, or some shortness of breath. These sensations are all related to the medication and are not dangerous. You will only receive the infusion for a couple of minutes, and the symptoms resolve quickly after the IV has been stopped.

Reginald's angiogram revealed that he had two blockages in two separate coronary arteries, both about 60 percent blocked. Since his blockages fell into the intermediate category, his cardiologist felt it would be important to conduct the FFR test. Reginald felt a little burning for about five minutes, but he had no problems tolerating the test. The FFR test showed that the blockages in both arteries caused only minimal impairment of blood flow. Thus Reginald's doctor determined that medication alone would be the best treatment.

Another blockage test, *intravascular ultrasound* (IVUS), can be conducted to determine whether a blockage is restricting blood flow. IVUS is frequently used for evaluating intermediate blockages. The test involves a tiny ultrasound probe that is so small it fits inside the coronary arteries! This allows doctors to visualize the inside of the blood vessels and determine the exact amount of plaque buildup.

Q U E S T I O N **18** ─────────

Brian, an electrical engineer, was fascinated to learn as many technical details as he could about the steps taken by his medical team to save his life when he had a heart attack. Therefore, after he learned about the diagnostic angiogram (Question 13), he wanted to find out more about angioplasty—the corrective aspect of the procedure. Since the angiogram and angioplasty had been done as an emergency procedure to save his life, Brian had not had an opportunity prior to the heart attack to understand how angioplasty worked. Now that he is beginning to feel healthy again, he wants to know more. The question he wants answered now is . . .

How does a coronary angioplasty work?

THE BOTTOM LINE

Angioplasty is the name of the treatment used to open a blockage that has been found during an angiogram. The word *angio* means "vessels," and *plasty* means "opening with a balloon." Prior to the invention of stents, angioplasty (known as *balloon angioplasty*) was a way to treat a coronary blockage by inflating a tiny balloon inside the blockage in order to open it. After the blockage had been opened by the balloon, the balloon was removed and nothing was left inside the blood vessel. Over the last fifteen years this procedure has greatly evolved, because now, after a balloon has been used to open the blockage, a stent is left inside the vessel to prop it open. Most people still refer to the procedure as angioplasty even though the technical term is now *percutaneous coronary intervention* (PCI). The change of name reflects the many different options to treating a blockage other than balloon angioplasty. In fact, balloon angioplasty is only rarely used now and is nicknamed POBA (plain old balloon angioplasty).

How does PCI actually work?

Under most circumstances, PCI is performed immediately after an angiogram reveals a significant blockage (see Question 13) during the same procedure. The doctor is able to use the same access tube for taking pictures and then for conducting the angioplasty. This is especially likely when a patient is brought to the hospital due to a heart attack, and the procedure is conducted to save his or her life, as was the case with Brian. He remembers learning that angiography (the angiogram) is when the doctor takes pictures (images) of the blood vessels in order to find the blockages. There are circumstances, however, when it is necessary to separate the two procedures (which is normal, acceptable medical practice). One reason for this might be that some facilities conduct only angiograms but not angioplasty.

Another reason that a medical team may want to do the angioplasty separately is that the angiogram may reveal that the blockage is very complex, and the doctor wants to analyze the results of the angiogram to determine the best course of treatment.

Several steps make up a coronary angioplasty, but none of these steps are complicated. The full sequence of the angioplasty procedure is shown in Figure 8.

1. The first step is very similar to the first part of an angiogram. A catheter (tube) is moved through the arteries and placed at the origin of the coronary artery (the blood vessel supplying blood to the heart). This catheter is slightly larger than the one used for an angiogram, but it is still very tiny. This slight increase in the size of the catheter is to accommodate the equipment that must travel through the tube.

2. Next, a thin wire only slightly thicker than a hair, with a very soft tip, is steered through the catheter toward the blockage and then through the blockage and positioned in the artery downstream of the blockage. This wire serves as a rail for the procedure much as train tracks guide a train.

3. A balloon is moved through the catheter along the wire to the blockage itself. Balloons come in different diameters and lengths (all very tiny). Your doctor will choose the one that best fits your blood vessel and the blockage.

4. Once the balloon is in place inside the blockage, it is inflated in order to crack the plaque of the blockage. The balloon remains inflated for thirty seconds to one minute. It is then released.

5. During this part of the procedure (and all those following), contrast dye is periodically injected in order to take images of your blood flow to evaluate each step of the procedure and to determine the next best step.

6. Once the blockage has been properly opened, the balloon is removed from the blockage and removed from the blood vessel and body.

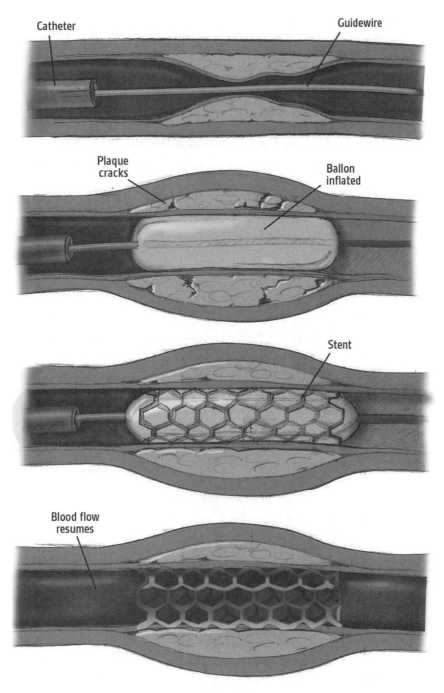

Figure 8

7. Another balloon with a stent mounted on top is introduced into the catheter. The stent is very thin and flexible and actually crimped onto the balloon. The flexible shape of the stent helps it move through the blood vessel. This is important, because when a vessel has been hardened by plaque, the stent's journey can be challenging.

8. Once the balloon and stent are inside the blockage, the balloon is inflated, which causes the stent to expand. The pressure of the balloon's inflation pushes the stent (which looks like a miniature metal scaffold) into the wall of the blood vessel. The stent pushes aside the plaque, moving it into the wall of the vessel, thus propping open the artery. The stent remains in place inside the coronary artery at the site of the blockage.

9. Once the stent is fully expanded, the balloon is deflated and removed.

10. Sometimes a third balloon is introduced to further expand (stretch) the stent to ensure that the plaque has been fully pushed aside.

11. Once the cardiologist is satisfied that the blockage has been adequately opened and that the stent is in the right place, the wire inside the coronary artery is removed. Final pictures are taken to confirm that the procedure has accomplished its job.

THE NITTY GRITTY

How does the balloon break through the hardened plaque?

A good question—with an interesting answer! In order for a coronary balloon to break through the hardened plaque of a blockage, very high pressure is used to inflate it. Typical pressures are between 10 and 20 atmospheres. In comparison, a car tire is inflated at around 2 atmospheres. But don't worry. A coronary balloon is extremely durable in order to withstand such pressure.

I always thought that angioplasty is like Roto-Rooter. Is that true?

Roto-Rooter was invented in the early 1930s by Samuel Blanc to solve the problem of clogged drains. Blanc designed a cable with sharp rotating blades that could be pushed through drains to cut tree roots out of sewer lines, eliminating the need to dig out the lines. The more modern-day Roto-Rooter (and similar) systems use chemicals to dissolve clogs in drains and restore drainage.

The concept of a coronary blockage is somewhat similar to a clogged drain, although the method used for clearing the "pipe" is quite different from a Roto-Rooter. Most people would not want sharp rotating blades or toxic chemicals inside their blood vessels! Interestingly, though, there are some medical tools somewhat similar to a Roto-Rooter that are occasionally used to clear blockages. These tools are used when simply moving the plaque isn't enough. As we discussed above, plaque is not removed from the artery, but rather displaced or pushed into the wall of the blood vessel. In unusual circumstances, when the hardening of a blood vessel is excessive, a stent might get stuck by the plaque inside an artery before it gets to the blockage. When this happens, a device called a Rotablator—a tool similar to a dentist's drill—is used to break up the calcification in the artery so the stent can move on to the blockage. The Rotablator might also be used when the plaque inside the blockage is so hard that even the strongest balloon cannot open it up. It is important to remember, however, that with the advancements in stent technology, this device is rarely used.

Is it possible to treat multiple blockages at the same time?

Yes, in fact, it is common for multiple blockages to be treated during the same procedure, although your doctor will repair one blockage at a time before moving on to the next one. It is not unusual to have multiple blockages in the same vessel and to receive multiple stents in that vessel, lined up one next to the other. If more than one vessel has a critical blockage, it is possible for multiple blockages to be treated in different vessels. Most doctors will limit the number of blockages treated during a procedure because this reduces the risk of using too much radiation and too much contrast dye (which could cause kidney damage). If after your angioplasty procedure you still have untreated blockages that require attention, your doctor will schedule a return visit for you a few weeks later to have another angioplasty procedure.

Q U E S T I O N **19**

For two months Michael has been taking medications exactly as his doctor prescribed for him: a blood thinner, a cholesterol lowering medication, and blood pressure medication. He has been trying to lose weight. Although Michael's wife, Dorothy, is cooking much more health-ily, he can't seem to stop himself from eating the forbidden foods (his favorite is a roast beef sandwich with mayo from a local deli). He feels guilty and knows that this—plus the cookies he sneaks at night—are not good for him, but he doesn't seem to have the willpower to stop. He also has not made it back to the gym, because he's afraid that the pain in his chest will come back if he starts to exercise. The bottom line is that Michael hasn't lost any weight. To make matters worse, last week he felt the pain in his chest again while walking upstairs at the end of the day.

This time Michael made an appointment with his cardiologist right away, expecting the worst. After seeing Michael, the doctor recom-mended that he have an angiogram. The doctor explained that since Michael's chest pain had returned, despite taking the medication, there was a good chance that he had a blockage in need of intervention.

Michael was worried about how the angiogram would feel, but he found it to be only a little stressful. The results of the angiogram revealed that he had a significant blockage requiring angioplasty. Since Michael's angiogram had been conducted at a hospital that does not support angioplasty procedures, he was transferred to a different facility for the procedure.

Now, Michael is really worried! He wishes that he had spent the last few months doing more to improve his health and lose weight. Michael's doctor tried to explain the science behind angioplasty and stents, but Michael doesn't really want to know too much about what might happen inside his body. The only thing he really wants to know is . . .

How will I feel during this procedure?

THE BOTTOM LINE

In many ways, what you experience and how you may feel during an angioplasty are similar to the way you feel when you have an angiogram. In fact, the first part—the preparation and the beginning of the procedure—is identical. Therefore, you should reread the beginning of Question 14 to remind yourself about how you will be prepped before you are brought into the procedure room.

Once in the procedure room, the first part of the experience is again identical to an angiogram. In fact, the first part of the angioplasty is an angiogram, even if you have had one previously. You will be placed on an x-ray table with a hard surface, but most people tolerate it with no problem. The room may be quite cold because this prevents the equipment from overheating. Don't hesitate to ask for a blanket or two to keep you warm.

Once you are settled on the table, you will be mildly sedated but not necessarily asleep, certainly not unconscious the way you would be with general anesthesia. At any point, if you are uncomfortable or feeling pain, you should tell the doctor so he or she can administer more sedation and pain medication. However, if you feel fine, don't ask for more, because it is not necessary for you to fall asleep.

Once you have been sedated, either your groin area or your wrist will be numbed with a local anesthetic and then a tube (known as a sheath) will be inserted into the area. This, too, is much like the steps taken to perform an angiogram, so if you want to, you can read more about this in Question 14. As you learned in Question 18, the sheath used for angioplasty is slightly larger than the one used for an angiogram because it has to accommodate the equipment used in the procedure, whereas the tube used in an angiogram need only accommodate the x-ray dye.

Michael was relieved to learn he would not feel any difference even though the tube is slightly larger.

Remember, since there are no nerves inside blood vessels, you will not feel any catheters moving inside your body.

Before the angioplasty is conducted, the coronary arteries are imaged using an angiogram. Even if you have had an angiogram before, and this is to be an elective (scheduled) angioplasty, the first part of the procedure will include exactly the same steps taken to perform an angiogram. You can refer back to Question 14 for the details.

The main difference between an angiogram and an angioplasty is that the angioplasty takes more time to perform, which means that you will be on the table and sedated for a longer period of time. An angiogram typically takes about thirty minutes to complete, while an angioplasty will add another thirty to sixty minutes to the procedure. The actual length of the procedure will depend upon a number of factors: where is the blockage? how easy or difficult is it to open the blockage? how many blockages are to be treated during the procedure? You shouldn't compare your procedure to that of someone else. Each person, doctor, and procedure is unique.

A complex angioplasty procedure can take up to two hours, and it is extremely important for you to remain very still throughout the procedure. You shouldn't move your arms, because this could contaminate the sterile field, which would expose you to potential infection. In addition, any movement could cause the catheter to move, which might disrupt the procedure. If you find that you are becoming uncomfortable lying on the table for this length of time, you should ask for additional sedation and pain medication.

During the angioplasty you may develop some chest discomfort or chest pressure. During Michael's angioplasty, he experienced the same discomfort he had felt when he was exercising on the treadmill. The doctor explained that this is normal. As each of the balloons (the first one and then the second one with the stent) is fully inflated inside the blockage, it temporarily cuts off the blood flow to the heart muscle, which causes discomfort. Since the balloon is inflated for thirty seconds to one minute, chest discomfort resolves quite rapidly. Under most circumstances the pain is mild and tolerable. But if you feel pain, don't hesitate to ask for pain medication.

As part of an angioplasty, your doctor may administer medication through the catheter. The most commonly used medication during this procedure is nitroglycerin, which enlarges the coronary blood vessels and prevents them from going into spasm. Nitroglycerin, however, does not work specifically on these blood vessels. Once inside your body, it will also enlarge the blood vessels in your brain, which causes a headache for some people. This headache is not typically serious, and it will end within a few minutes. If the headache does not go away or if it gets worse, you should tell your doctor immediately.

Michael's procedure took about ninety minutes. He received two stents in one artery. Michael asked for additional sedation when he started to feel very uncomfortable lying on the table. He also asked for more pain medication for a headache. Overall, Michael felt that the procedure was manageable, although he was relieved when it was over.

THE NITTY GRITTY

What causes the chest pain during the angioplasty (or during exercise)?

Your heart muscle is constantly pumping blood. It never rests! Therefore, it needs a constant supply of oxygen and nutrients. These nutrients are supplied by the blood that is pumped into the heart. When this supply is interrupted (by the balloon, by a heart attack, or because exercise places too great a demand on a partially blocked vessel), and the demand outweighs the supply, most people (but not all) develop chest pain. During angioplasty, this pain is temporary and will typically resolve when the balloon is deflated. However, don't forget that the balloon is used at least twice during the procedure (sometimes more if the blockage is stubborn). So you may feel discomfort with each inflation.

Since it is normal to get chest pain during the procedure, should I worry if I don't feel anything?

Certainly not. Some people do not experience discomfort when they have critical blockages *or* even while having a heart attack. Similarly, not everyone will have chest discomfort during an angioplasty, especially since the balloon is inflated for only a short time.

What if my chest discomfort does not resolve?

Almost half of all angioplasty patients will have some chest discomfort that persists for a few hours or even up to a day after the procedure.[12] This is thought to be due to *stretch pain* when the balloon and stent prop open the blockage and slightly stretch the artery. This discomfort is usually benign (of no medical significance), sort of like a muscle ache. Nevertheless, you should *always* tell your doctor if you develop chest pain after the procedure or if your chest pain does not resolve, because it is possible for this pain to be an indication of a problem with the stent (see Question 22 for possible complications).

20

Rosa's recovery from her heart attack has been a little slow. She still doesn't feel quite like herself, and she can't help worrying about her long-term health. It also seems strange to Rosa that she has little bits of metal inside her body, namely, the stents that saved her life. She thinks about those stents a lot, often wondering to herself . . .

My doctor placed a stent in my coronary artery. What exactly is a stent?

THE BOTTOM LINE

A stent is a tiny metal tube designed much like a rolled-up chain-link fence (see an illustration of a closed, not yet deployed stent on a balloon and an opened, deployed stent in Figure 9). The first stents were made of stainless steel. Stainless steel is a very strong metal, and it has good radial strength (the ability to open a blockage and keep it open despite the compressing force exerted by the blood vessel and the blockage). Since stainless steel is stiff and inflexible, it was sometimes difficult to move stents through the artery and position them in the blockage. Newer stents are made from metal alloys like cobalt-chromium. They are much thinner and more flexible than the original stainless steel stents but still have excellent radial strength. This is important because the main advantage of placing a stent,

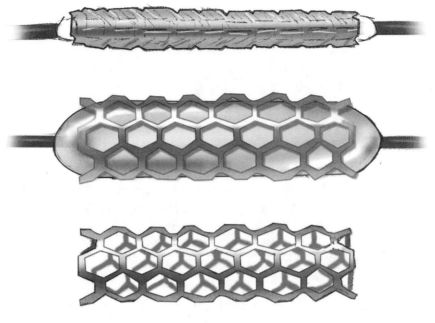

Figure 9

rather than simply treating the blockage with balloon angioplasty alone, is that the stent stops the vessel from collapsing (known as *vessel recoil*) after the balloon is removed.

Where does the stent end up?

As the stent opens, it pushes the blocking plaque into the wall of the blood vessel. Once a stent is in place, it cannot be removed (see Question 18 for more details), because the force of the expanding balloon pushes the stent into the wall of the blood vessel, embedding it there *permanently*.

It is permanent because, over time, the original plaque of the blockage remains behind the stent (pushed there by the stent as the balloon expanded it) and healthy tissue forms over the stent, covering it fully, like a wall. In fact, if you had a camera inside the blood vessel, eventually you would no longer be able to tell where the stent was placed (see Figure 10), because it looks identical to the rest of the vessel.

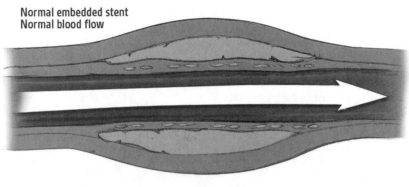

Normal embedded stent
Normal blood flow

Figure 10

Is it necessary to leave the stent in the wall of the artery as a permanent scaffold?

This is a good question, and from a medical perspective the answer is somewhat unclear. It is theoretically possible that if a stent remains inside a vessel for some time, it might allow the vessel to remodel and become stronger so that it would not collapse, even if the stent was removed. Research under way is testing a bioabsorbable stent. This type of stent is placed like a regular stent, providing the initial support necessary to keep the vessel open, but the stent is made from a material that disintegrates over time so that the stent disappears from your body within a year or two. It is too soon to know whether this type of stent holds any advantages over a regular one.

Are there any risks with stents?

There are, in fact, two possible complications associated with stents.

1. **In-stent restenosis.** As you now know, it is part of the healing process for the metal stent eventually to be completely covered

over with tissue. Sometimes, however, the body produces too much tissue inside the stent. This is similar to the way a cut may heal with a keloid (excessive scar tissue), causing the healed scar to be raised rather than flat. When this happens with a stent, it is called *in-stent restenosis*, which means re-blockage of the stent (Figure 11). The symptoms of in-stent restenosis are similar to the symptoms of the original blockage (chest pressure with exertion), and when this happens, another angioplasty procedure may be necessary.

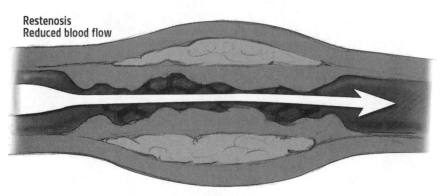

**Restenosis
Reduced blood flow**

Figure 11

In-stent restenosis occurs about 10–30 percent of the time, or in one to three people out of ten, and depends upon individual risk factors. Patients who have diabetes are at increased risk for this complication, and it is also more likely to occur when a stent is placed in a very small vessel or when a very long or multiple stents are placed in a vessel.

To reduce the risk of in-stent restenosis, drug-eluting stents were developed. These stents are coated with a medication that prevents excess scar tissue from forming. In Questions 20 and 21, we will discuss in-stent restenosis and drug-eluting stents in much greater detail.

2. **Stent thrombosis.** Stent thrombosis is a more serious potential complication in which a blood clot forms inside the stent, much like the development of a heart attack. It can, in fact, cause a

heart attack (Figure 12). Fortunately, this is a very rare event, occurring in only 1–2 percent (one to two people out of one hundred) of stent recipients. The symptoms of stent thrombosis are the same as those of a heart attack (see Question 1). Therefore if, after receiving a stent, you suspect that you may be having a heart attack, don't assume it is nothing. Call 911 immediately and follow the instructions outlined in Question 1. You will minimize your risk of stent thrombosis if you take your medications exactly as prescribed, especially the blood-thinning medication (usually aspirin along with either Plavix, Effient, or Brilinta)

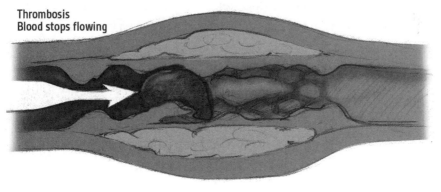

**Thrombosis
Blood stops flowing**

Figure 12

THE NITTY GRITTY

Ask most knowledgeable people to define a stent, and they will say that it is a tube placed into a heart artery during an angioplasty to open a blockage and keep the artery open. But ask a urologist what a stent is, and he or she will respond that it is used to replace a damaged ureter or other natural tube. A radiologist will inform you that a stent is a device used for drainage during a procedure. Medical doctors in different disciplines will have their own definitions of a stent, and in fact, the word *stent* can be used to describe several completely different medical devices.

The word *stent* comes from its creator, Charles Stent (1807–1885), an English dentist who invented a compound to produce dentures. This compound was subsequently used for many other purposes, including skin grafts and developing hollow tubes. Charles Stent won great recognition when he suggested using his material to coat the underwater transatlantic cable, which had broken several times as a result of corrosion by seawater. His accomplishments led to an appointment in 1855 as Dentist to the Royal Household.

Most stents start out as a solid, hollow tube. The openings (a lattice-like effect) are then created with laser cuts, although some newer stents are braided from individual thin metal wires. This design is intended to keep the stent as flexible as possible, which is critical because the coronary arteries have many twists and turns, and an inflexible tube would not be able to make the turns necessary to traverse an artery and reach a blockage.

There are many design variations used to create stents, and all very similar in their ability to do the intended job: move the stent smoothly through the artery, open the blockage, and keep it open. The stent design distinguishes one stent provider from another. There are small differences between stents, but basically the type of stent you receive depends largely on your doctor's preference.

QUESTION **21** ────────

Brian continues to become more and more knowledgeable about his heart disease and the ways he can improve his odds of living a long and healthy life. His wife, kids, and friends admire the way he has so dramatically changed his lifestyle since having a heart attack. In fact, recently, Brian was offered the opportunity to write a short article for a website about how it felt to survive the heart attack. The article is meant to educate others about heart attacks and angioplasty from a patient's perspective. Brian feels confident that he will be able to write a terrific article, but there is one thing that he is still not sure about . . .

My doctor said I was given a drug-coated stent. Is that better?

THE BOTTOM LINE

For most patients the answer is *yes*. A drug-coated (drug-eluting) stent is a better choice. In order to understand whether it is the best choice for you requires a bit of knowledge about your body.

When a person receives any stent, the blood vessel must adjust to this tiny metal intrusion. Miraculously, it is able to do so, starting to heal almost immediately by growing tissue around the stent much as a scar heals on a skin wound. The goal is for your body to grow enough tissue that the stent is fully covered and not exposed to the constant flow of blood, but not too much tissue, because this will block the blood flow again. As we described in Question 20, when this happens, it is called in-stent restenosis, and you are likely to feel chest pain just as you probably did when you first had a blockage.

Medication-coated (drug-eluting) stents are specifically designed to reduce the possibility of tissue overgrowth. In fact, in-stent restenosis occurs in about 10 to 30 percent of patients who receive regular metal stents (also known as bare-metal stents). When a drug-eluting stent is placed, the chance of restenosis is reduced to less than 10 percent!

How does a drug-eluting stent work?

The stent itself is identical to a bare-metal stent (see Question 20), and the medication that inhibits the formation of scar tissue is bonded to the metal of the stent. This medication is released over time (usually a few weeks to a few months), and it substantially reduces tissue growth or scar formation inside the stent, thus reducing the chances of in-stent restenosis. It does not reduce it to zero, but it reduces the chances of restenosis to less than 10 percent.

The medication causes the blood vessel to heal more slowly around the stent than it otherwise would heal. This slowed healing process requires the patient to be on a blood-thinning medication for a longer period of time than a person receiving a noncoated stent. Therefore, in order to be a candidate for a drug-eluting stent, the patient must be medically able to take the required blood-thinning medication (aspirin and another blood thinner like Plavix, Effient, or Brillinta) for at least a year after the angioplasty procedure. If your doctor determines that you are not able to take this medication for at least a year, uninterrupted, then a noncoated stent is probably a better choice for you.

If you receive a drug-eluting stent, it is very important to take your medications as prescribed. Do *not* stop taking blood thinners without medical clearance from your cardiologist. If you have a bad reaction to a medication, speak to your doctor immediately or go to an emergency room.

THE NITTY GRITTY

Since drug-eluting stents causes the blood vessel to heal more slowly, the metal of the stent is exposed to the blood flowing through the vessel for a longer period of time before fully healing. The longer the metal is exposed to the blood, the greater the possibility that the blood will recognize the metal as a foreign object. If this happens, blood platelets (parts of the blood) might, in very rare cases, attach to the metal stent, forming a blood clot inside the stent, called a stent thrombosis (see Question 20). This thrombosis is a sudden blockage that occurs with no warning, similar to a heart attack. It prevents blood flow, which could cause a heart attack. Taking blood thinners like aspirin plus another blood thinner significantly reduces the likelihood of a clot being developing. This is why it is essential for a potential drug-eluting stent candidate to be able to take blood thinners for at least a year after the stent procedure.

Even if you do everything you are supposed to do, there are other risk factors for stent thrombosis, including

- The size of the treated vessel (the smaller the diameter, the higher the likelihood)
- The length of the blockage (longer blockages require longer stents, and these have higher rates of thrombosis)
- The need for multiple overlapping stents (the more stents, the greater the chance of blood clot formation)
- Diabetes

Drug-coated stents are a remarkable innovation, but they are not for everyone. If you cannot take blood thinners for the prescribed year due to bleeding problems, or if you have a surgery or major procedure scheduled in the near future, you may not be a candidate for a drug-coated stent. Under these circumstances it may be better to use a nonmedicated stent. Be sure to share all your health information with your cardiologist because he or she will need this in order to make a decision that is best for your health.

QUESTION **22**

Michael, a self-proclaimed worrier, is relieved that the angioplasty was not very uncomfortable. He got through it by focusing on the positives (how it was going to help him) and none of the potential negatives. But now that it is over, he can't help thinking about what could have gone wrong. He's also concerned about possible risks should he need to have this procedure again. Michael can't wait for his next cardiology appointment so that he can ask his doctor . . .

Can anything go wrong during the angioplasty procedure?

THE BOTTOM LINE

Every invasive procedure has some amount of risk. Specific risks depend on the particular procedure. When it comes to angioplasty, the risks are relatively small because the procedure has been perfected over the last forty years. Technological advances, medical training and experience, and the right combination of medications make it extraordinarily safe. Angioplasty is performed over one million times a year worldwide with very low rates of complications or adverse events.

That being said, there are specific risks associated with angioplasty, which we discuss below, but the degree of risk differs from person to person, depending on individual risk factors. This means that your risk varies based on your conditions as well as the particular blockage to be treated.

The main factors that increase risk for complications during angioplasty include

1. Advanced age (the older you are, the more likely you are to experience complications)
2. Female gender (while the research isn't conclusive, this may be because women have smaller blood vessels, which increases the risk for vascular complications)
3. Diabetes (which can damage blood vessels)
4. Chronic kidney failure
5. Large amounts of hardened plaque (more difficult to treat)
6. Specific location of the blockage within the coronary arteries

The more of these risk factors you have, the greater your risks for complications.

Now that you understand the risk factors that increase the chance for complications, it is important to remember that, even with some of these risk factors present, this is still a very safe procedure. For example, if your particular risk factors double your risk of a complication, in reality you increase your risk from very, very small to slightly greater (still a very small risk). It is comforting to know that the overall rate of life-threatening complications (even if you have some of these risk factors) is in most cases *still* less than 1 percent. This means that ninety-nine out of one hundred people do very well. This is the reason that angioplasty procedures are performed so frequently with such success all around the world.

What are the possible complications?

Reading through the possible complications might make you anxious, but keep in mind that all these complications are very, very rare and it is unlikely that you will experience any of them.

Bleeding

In the 2–3 percent of cases that bleeding occurs, it is often local bleeding, which means that it is found at the site where the access tube is inserted (typically in the groin). This might be uncomfortable, but it is life threatening, and there is even less risk when the wrist is used. There is some new research that indicates that bleeding might be associated with a greater risk of dying, even one year after the procedure, which is part of the reason that there is an increased interest by cardiologists to use the wrist as the access site (see more about access sites in Questions 10 and 13).

Since the catheter crosses through the abdominal cavity, there is a small chance of injury, potentially resulting in bleeding. This is called a *retroperitoneal bleed*, which can be very serious because a great deal of blood can pool in the belly. This complication can often be treated with a blood transfusion, although sometimes it requires emergency abdominal surgery and on occasion can be fatal.

Heart attack

There is a small chance that someone might suffer a heart attack during an angioplasty. This type of a heart attack occurs when a very small piece of plaque becomes dislodged during the procedure and then blocks a capillary (a tiny vessel in the heart). These vessels are too small to be visualized by the coronary angiography, and most of the time there are no signs or symptoms during the procedure of this tiny heart attack. It is only detected by the blood work after the procedure and is rarely associated with any damage to the heart or any other problems. Large heart attacks are rare, and fatal heart attacks are even more uncommon.

Stroke

The aorta is the main blood vessel in your body. It exits the heart and supplies blood to the entire body. The aorta is the main highway in the body, connecting the entire system of arteries in your body. Sometimes plaque builds up in the aorta just as it does in other blood vessels. Stroke, a very rare complication, occasionally occurs when some plaque breaks loose from the aorta when the catheter travels from the groin or wrist toward the heart.

Reaction to the dye (contrast material)

Complications related to the use of dye are not specific to having an angiogram or angioplasty. It can occur during any procedure that uses dye. For example, this is the same contrast material that is used during CT scans, so the same risks apply. There are two potential risks associated with the contrast dye used during an angioplasty (or angiogram).

The first potential problem is damage to the kidneys caused by toxic effects that the dye may have (more on this in The Nitty Gritty). Most people tolerate the dye without any problem, though. However, preexisting kidney damage or long-standing diabetes may place the kidneys at risk for further damage. When damage occurs, kidneys usually heal themselves, but sometimes a kidney injury can be permanent and, in worst-case scenarios, can even lead to the need for dialysis.

The second potential complication is an allergic reaction to the contrast dye. This might cause itching, hives, swelling of eyelids or tongue, or difficulty swallowing or breathing. It can even result in anaphylaxis, which is a potentially fatal reaction in which you cannot breathe, your blood pressure drops, and you go into shock. If you have had contrast dye in the past, resulting in any reaction (no matter how minor), *you must inform your doctor before the procedure.* This is extremely important, because if you are allergic to the dye, your doctor must reassess the importance of the procedure, given the risks. If your doctor decides to proceed with the angioplasty, you will be able to receive medication beforehand to avoid a potentially fatal complication. You should also be sure to tell your doctor if you have any allergies to any other medications. Also, if you experience any of the symptoms described above during the procedure, tell your health care team right away!

Injury to other blood vessels

In very rare circumstances injury may occur to other arteries or even to the aorta. This could lead to a tear or rupturing of a vessel, which can lead to bleeding. The precise treatment for such an unusual complication depends on each unique situation.

THE NITTY GRITTY

What is the snowplow effect?

As you can see from Figure 1 (in chapter 1), there are many small blood vessels branching from the major coronary arteries. When a stent is placed in one of the major arteries (or a large branch), it typically blocks (or jails) some of the smaller branches. This is typically not problematic because the stent is an open lattice (see Figure 9) through which blood can still move into the smaller branches. However, it is possible for the stent procedure to push plaque into one of the branches, much as a snowplow blocks driveways as it moves the snow aside. If this happens, it is often possible to reopen the side branch using a small balloon, but in some instances, the vessel may be too small to open, which could lead to a small heart attack.

Another complication that might lead to heart attack is a tear of the artery when the balloon is inflated to open the blockage. This happens quite frequently, and most of the time the tear is small and does not obstruct or decrease blood flow in the coronary artery, therefore it does not impair blood flow to the heart muscle. Sometimes, however, the tear in the blood vessel is extensive and reduces or even completely blocks the flow of blood. If this happens, the heart muscle does not receive an adequate supply of blood, much like a heart attack. Fortunately, most of the time, your interventional cardiologist can fix the problem quickly by placing a stent at the location of the tear. This stent not only props open the blockage but also tacks down the tear, reestablishing the blood flow to the heart. If this is accomplished with relative speed, there is typically no damage to the heart at all. In very rare circumstances, where it is not possible to place a stent and reopen the blood vessel, you may suffer a heart attack. Sometimes this leads to an emergency bypass surgery (more on bypass surgery in Question 24).

Is it possible to prevent kidney damage caused by the dye?

After contrast dye has been introduced to the body in order to take pictures of the blood vessels, the dye must be eliminated from the body. It is the job of the kidneys to eliminate the dye along with other impurities. An accumulation of dye in the kidneys can hurt the kidneys. This damage, caused by the contrast dye, is called *contrast-induced nephropathy*.

The most effective way to prevent this damage is to flush the dye from the kidneys with lots of intravenous fluids. This is the reason that you will usually receive IV fluids before and after the procedure. There is some debate as to whether certain fluids are better than others, but the bottom line is that more fluids are better, no matter which one is chosen! There is also one medication often recommended for those people at risk for developing kidney damage (those people who already have some kidney damage or who have diabetes). If you have ever been received this medication (it's called N-acetylcysteine or Mucomyst), you won't forget it, because it smells like ammonia.

Q U E S T I O N **23** ⎯⎯⎯⎯⎯⎯

Rosa's health is continuing to improve with each passing day, and she feels very happy and grateful that she was able to survive the heart attack. She is taking all her medications regularly, and she is doing her best to follow her doctor's directions. Rosa is not usually the type of person who is curious about the details of her health, but this time, as the days and weeks go by, she keeps thinking about the stent she received, without which she might not be alive today.

"It's like a miracle!" she tells her friends every time she shares her story. Now, Rosa really wants to know . . .

Does a stent actually help stop a heart attack?

THE BOTTOM LINE

Yes, it does. There have been many studies that have looked at this question, and the majority of experts agree that the most effective way to treat a heart attack is by performing an angioplasty and placing a stent. That being said, *the most important factor in successful treatment is to receive the angioplasty as early as possible.*

Current guidelines recommend that when you have a heart attack, an emergency angioplasty should be performed *within ninety minutes* of your arrival in the emergency room, no matter what time of day or night you have the heart attack, as long as the hospital is equipped to perform emergency angioplasties. Most hospitals that offer twenty-four-hour, seven-day-a-week emergency angioplasty are able to achieve this goal of treatment within ninety minutes of arrival unless there are other complicating factors. In fact, you might be interested to learn that, over the last ten years, doctors have decreased the amount of time it takes them to open a blockage, from three hours to one hour.

This is great, but in reality it only addresses half the problem. This is because the heart attack does not occur *when* you arrive at the ER but sometime prior. The majority of people wait too long before calling for help. In fact, scientific studies indicate that most people wait an average of two hours before calling an ambulance. This is a *big* problem because the *sooner* you call for help, the *sooner* you can receive treatment. The more quickly you receive treatment, the better your chances are for minimizing the damage to your heart from the heart attack.

Although she was uncomfortable, Rosa waited several hours before going to the emergency room. The angioplasty did save her life, but had she gone sooner, she would likely have had less damage to her heart and perhaps a shorter recovery. In some cases, waiting as long as Rosa waited could result in someone dying before reaching the ER.

**If you think you may be having a heart attack,
don't wait to see what happens. Call 911 immediately!**

Receiving treatment quickly for a heart attack is *so* important that the American Heart Association and the American College of Cardiology have an ongoing educational campaign based on the idea that "Time Is Muscle." The message of this campaign is that the most important factor in surviving a heart attack is *minimizing the time from the onset of symptoms* (the beginning of the heart attack) *until the blockage is opened with angioplasty* and *blood flow to the heart muscle is reestablished.* When delay is minimized, heart muscle is preserved and lives are saved.

Okay, I get it. But why is it so important to open the blockage as soon as possible?

As you know from Question 2, a heart attack occurs when a small blood clot attaches itself to a partial blockage in a blood vessel, suddenly and completely blocking the blood flow in the vessel. At this point, oxygen and other nutrients no longer reach the part of the heart muscle that receives blood from that vessel. If the blockage is opened within a certain period of time (usually two to four hours), the blood flow will be restored and there is minimal or no damage to the heart. However, if the blockage remains in place for too long, that part of the heart muscle dies, which causes *permanent* damage to the heart. This is just another way of explaining that it is critical to call for an ambulance as soon as possible if you even think you might be having a heart attack.

What are the treatment options?

The goal in treating a heart attack is to dissolve the blood clot that is blocking blood flow and reestablish the blood supply to the heart muscle. As you now know, angioplasty is the best way of doing this. Another very effective treatment (although it won't replace an angioplasty) is to take medication that dissolves blood clots. You might be surprised to know that one such medication is over-the-counter aspirin. Therefore, if you think you are having a heart attack, *you should* take aspirin *immediately* while waiting for the ambulance. In fact, if you have any risk factors for having a heart attack, it is a good idea to keep a supply of aspirin at home and in your car. This is not a step to take if you are allergic to aspirin or if you have had any serious reactions to it in the past, such as internal bleeding.

Another effective mediation, sometimes given in the emergency room, is called a clot buster. This medication is frequently administered at hospitals that are not equipped to perform emergency angioplasty procedures and when the next-closest capable hospital is too far away to achieve the ninety-minute goal of opening the blockage.

Although clot busters may sound like an easy treatment, they work only about half the time (a 50–60 percent success rate). This is the reason that angioplasty is a better treatment for heart attacks if it is available. During angioplasty, a blood clot can be extracted (sucked out) of the blood vessel and the blockage is propped open with a stent, which reestablishes blood flow to the heart muscle almost immediately. Angioplasty has a success rate of more than 90 percent, which is much better than the success rate of the clot-busting medication.

THE NITTY GRITTY

What if I can't get an emergency angioplasty?

Angioplasty procedures are primarily performed at larger hospitals because they have the technology and trained medical personnel. In reality, only a minority of people having heart attacks have access to such facilities in time to adequately treat heart attacks. Since it takes a certain amount of time to transfer a heart attack patient from a community hospital to a larger hospital that has the capability to perform angioplasty, the ninety-minute goal for having the angioplasty may be lost.

Currently only a minority of patients in the United States receive emergency angioplasty for a heart attack. According to recent statistics, this number has increased from less than 10 percent in 1994 to 20 percent in 2001[13] It is gratifying to know this number has doubled in less than ten years, however, it still means that fewer than 50 percent of patients have the benefit of the best possible treatment for a heart attack. If you find yourself having a heart attack at a facility that does not offer angioplasties, you will likely receive clot-busting medication, which is the next best treatment.

How much of a difference is there between hospitals?

A recent study known as the Global Utilization of Strategies to Open Occluded Arteries (GUSTO) IIb found that patients having a heart attack had a *relatively* higher mortality (death) rate at hospitals that are not capable of conducting angioplasties when compared to hospitals that do perform angioplasties.[14] This research has prompted more and more community hospitals to offer emergency angioplasty, even if they are not equipped to perform bypass surgery. There is some risk to this, because in rare circumstances a patient having an angioplasty might require emergency bypass surgery. However, ongoing research appears to show that, in this situation, the rewards (saving lives) outweigh the risks.

Q U E S T I O N

Diane was terribly upset when she found out that she had multiple blockages in her coronary arteries. And she felt even worse when her doctor revealed that so many blockages in multiple coronary arteries meant that she would be better off with bypass surgery than a stent procedure.

"Why me?" Diane cried to her best friend Evelyn. "So many people smoke, and nothing happens to them!"

"You're right," responded Evelyn, "but you also have a somewhat unfortunate family history. Your mom died of a heart attack in her fifties—there's nothing that you can do about that now. I've been your best friend for over thirty years, so I don't think that I'm out of line when I say that you probably should have stopped smoking many years ago in order to increase your chances of being healthy."

Diane nodded her head in agreement. She knew Evelyn was right.

"What exactly did the doctor say?" asked Evelyn.

"He told me that . . . "

My blockages cannot be fixed with a stent. I need bypass surgery. Then he told me what happens next . . .

THE BOTTOM LINE

Many (in fact, most) blockages can be treated with stents. Given the continuing improvement in stent technology, the introduction of drug-coated stents, and doctors' increasing experience, more and more patients can be treated with angioplasty rather than bypass surgery. However, certain types of blockages are better treated with bypass surgery. After you have a coronary angiogram, your doctor will best decide which treatment option is the best fit for your type of blockage or blockages.

When might I need bypass surgery?

The need for bypass surgery is determined by several factors:

- When there is a great deal of calcification (hardening), it might be very difficult to successfully place a stent, because the balloon won't be able to break through the hard calcification, especially when the blockage involves a large part of the blood vessel.

- When the repair of a blockage is particularly complex, there is risk of injury to the blood vessel. Performing a bypass reduces this risk.
- If there are multiple blockages, it may not be possible to place that many stents. In addition, when there are many blockages in a row, bypass surgery is able to get around all of them at the same time. The bypass is then sewn into the coronary artery downstream of the blockages.
- The location of a blockage is very important, because certain blockage locations actually make it more dangerous to place a stent than to have bypass surgery (more on this later).

Diane's coronary angiogram revealed that she had blockages in all of her major arteries as well as in some of the larger branches. Her cardiologist felt that far too many stents were needed to fix all the blockages. In addition, since Diane is diabetic, there is a somewhat greater chance that she would experience in-stent restenosis (recurrent blockages inside the stent). For these reasons he recommended that Diane have bypass surgery. Although Diane was shocked and upset about this, her doctor reassured her that bypass surgery has substantially improved in recent years and is much safer than Diane would have thought.

What exactly is bypass surgery?

The name—bypass—gives you a clue. A blockage is not treated directly, the way it is during an angioplasty procedure. Instead, the blockage is left alone and a new blood vessel (the bypass) is created around the blocked area (see Figure 13). You might imagine the blockage as a traffic jam on a major highway. Rather than clearing the traffic jam (performing an angioplasty), you redirect traffic onto another road that detours around the traffic jam, rejoining the major highway at a point beyond the jam (bypass surgery).

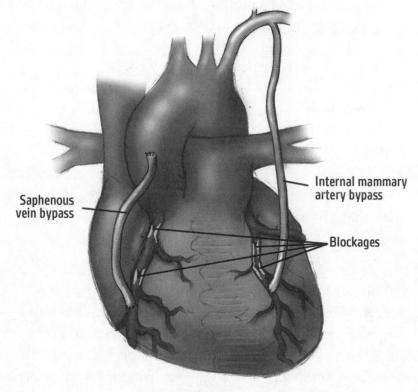

Internal mammary artery bypass

Saphenous vein bypass

Blockages

Figure 13

Unlike angioplasty, which is a procedure, bypass is major surgery. The surgery is performed under general anesthesia so the doctor can open your chest and attach the bypasses to the heart. Under most circumstances the chest is opened through the sternum (breastbone), in the middle of the chest. This provides good access to the heart, which is situated just underneath. After the surgery, the breastbone is splinted with wires before the chest is sutured closed. This surgery results in a scar down the middle of your chest.

While performing this surgery, most surgeons stop the heart and then restart it after the surgery has been completed. While the heart is stopped, it is not pumping blood to the rest of the body. Therefore, an artificial pump (called a heart-lung machine) is used to make sure that the body receives blood and oxygen throughout the surgery. While this might sound scary, it is a routine surgery that has been perfected over many years.

What is used to make the bypass?

The bypass comes from blood vessels in your own body! It is created from either an arterial graft (the bypass is made from an artery) or a venous graft (the bypass is made from a vein). The most commonly used bypass comes from an artery called the *internal mammary artery*. This artery is in the chest, and it supplies blood to the chest wall. This is the best blood vessel to use because the chest wall receives enough blood supply from other sources, so it is not a problem to divert this one and use it as a bypass graft to the heart. In addition, this is the most durable bypass, with the best longevity, so it is used in more than 90 percent of bypass cases.

Since many people require more than one bypass, other vessels may have to be used as well. When this is the case, your doctor will take a vein from your leg and move it to your heart. In this case, you will have a small scar on your leg in addition to the one on your chest.

How long is the recovery from bypass surgery?

When the surgery is completed with no complications, a bypass patient will stay in the hospital for five to seven days after the surgery. After being discharged from the hospital, some people will be moved to a cardiac rehabilitation center for another week or two before returning home. This rehabilitation helps the heart begin the healing process. In addition, the breastbone will be somewhat painful as it mends, and it can take one to two months to fully recover from this major surgery.

Diane's surgery was successful and she began to recover well. She experienced some chest pain when she took a deep breath (from the healing breastbone), but it was tolerable. Diane's doctor was con-cerned that she would not be able to take care of herself, due to her back problems and trouble moving around, so she did not go home directly after the surgery. Rather, she sent Diane to a rehabilitation center for two weeks. Diane had two sessions a day of rehab (exer-cise) and she met many people who, just like her, were recovering from heart disease. Evelyn came to visit her each day, and during one visit she was happy to see that Diane was receiving quite a bit of attention from a particularly sweet gentleman named Harry who had also had bypass surgery.

THE NITTY GRITTY

What if my heart does not restart after the bypass surgery?

This is the most pressing concern that most people have. In fact, it almost never happens except for extraordinary circumstances when the heart is very unhealthy before the surgery.

Of greater concern is that some people experience some degree of short-term memory loss after the surgery. This memory loss is attributed by some people to being on the heart-lung machine while the heart is stopped. Therefore this phenomenon is referred to as *pump head*. A great deal of research has been conducted on this phenomenon, but no conclusive results have been reached. In fact, most studies indicate that there is no difference in memory loss, regardless of whether the pump is used during bypass surgery. Some people do not believe that the memory loss is a real medical phenomenon.

Some surgeons offer the surgery off pump, which means that the heart is not stopped during surgery (so the pump is not needed). This definitely makes the surgery much more challenging, because the surgeon must suture the bypass onto the coronary artery while the heart is beating.

Can the surgery be done less invasively?

In some circumstances minimally invasive bypass surgery is possible. This requires only a small incision at the side of the chest, between the ribs, rather than breaking the breastbone. Since the breastbone is intact, recovery is much easier. However, this type of surgery is possible only when a single bypass is necessary. When multiple bypasses are needed, more of the heart must be exposed, and it is preferable to access the heart through the breastbone.

Diane had a quadruple bypass. What's that?

The number indicates the number of bypasses placed. Quadruple means four, which means that Diane had four bypasses placed in her heart. It is important to note that the surgery is not larger or more dangerous as the number increases. Therefore a quadruple bypass (four bypasses) is no more serious than a triple bypass (three bypasses). In other words, you should get as many bypasses as you require to treat as many blockages as possible. The only difference is that the surgery takes longer when more bypasses need to be done.

Can a bypass develop a blockage?

Yes, it can. Ten years marks the average amount of time that a bypass remains open before becoming blocked. Of course, *average* means that some bypasses become blocked within weeks and others stay open for thirty years. There are many factors that impact the rate at which a bypass will become blocked: the size of the coronary artery onto which the bypass is sutured, the amount of plaque in the vessel, the presence of other illnesses (like diabetes or kidney failure), and other factors associated with the surgery. Bypasses can also develop plaque buildup and blockages just like coronary arteries, therefore a bypass is not a "cure" for heart disease. It is still very important to live a heart-healthy life and to take your medications!

QUESTION **25** _____

Michael had his angioplasty procedure three days ago and is now recuperating at home. His wife, Dorothy, keeps telling him to relax and take it easy. She won't let him do anything for himself, and it is making him feel terribly helpless. In addition, when he's around his daughter Jessica, he often catches her giving him sad, worried looks. Michael doesn't like feeling sick or weak. He wants his situation to get better as soon as possible. He wonders . . .

When can I get back to my regular life?

THE BOTTOM LINE

One advantage of receiving a stent is that it is a *minimally* invasive procedure. This means that your recovery time is usually very short. As long as you don't have any complications, you can expect to go home on the same day as your procedure or the following day.

Michael left the hospital eight hours after his stent procedure.

Once you have been discharged after a stent procedure, there are very few precautions. If you experience chest pain or pressure from the blockage with strenuous activities, you should begin to feel better immediately. Most important is that you begin taking medications immediately after your discharge from the hospital and you continue to take them exactly as prescribed.

In addition to taking all your medications, for about a week you will need to take precautions to minimize any chance that the access site (the place in your groin or arm into which the catheter was inserted) will start bleeding. Your doctor will tell you to be careful to avoid putting pressure on the area or straining it. Activities to avoid (typically for about a week) include

- Lifting anything more than 20 to 30 pounds
- Strenuous exercise
- Weight lifting
- Some doctors recommend avoiding driving for one or two days after the procedure

Observing these limitations does not mean you cannot do anything. In fact, directly after surgery you are able to walk at a regular pace, use stairs, and sit or lie down as you have always done.

When is it safe to start exercising?

You might be anxious to get back to your regular exercise routine or to begin your new, healthier lifestyle as soon as possible. Therefore, you will be happy to know that most doctors recommend beginning exercise about a week after the procedure, by which time the insertion site should be healed. Before returning to or beginning an exercise schedule, you should check the access site (wrist or groin) to ensure there are no signs of continuous or recurrent bleeding at the site or any swelling in the area. If you notice any of these signs, call your doctor. Don't begin an exercise program until you are confident that you are fully healed and have medical clearance.

When is it safe to return to work?

The answer to this question depends on what type of work you do. If you have a sedentary job that does not require heavy lifting or strenuous activities, you should be able to return to work within a few days. If your job occasionally requires heavy lifting, be sure that someone else can help you out with this until you have medical clearance to lift heavy weights. If your job includes consistently strenuous activity or heavy lifting, you should talk to your doctor about when it is safe for you to return to work.

What about sex?

There is a great deal of controversy surrounding the safety of sexual intercourse for people with CAD. In fact, recently, the American Heart Association (AHA) released a statement to address the issue.[15] The recommendations in this statement are probably the most comprehensive to date and have been compiled by a group of experts in a range of fields including cardiology, exercise physiology, sexual counseling, and urology. The main takeaway is that *the risk of a heart attack is only very slightly increased during sexual activity and represents only a miniscule amount of a person's overall risk.* Therefore, for most people with CAD, it is safe to engage in sexual activity. The only patients who should refrain from sex are those with unstable heart disease or severe symptoms. These individuals should be assessed and stabilized with appropriate treatment before engaging in sexual activity.

Aside from receiving medical clearance to engage in sexual activity, it is important to note that many individuals with CAD experience anxiety or depression as a result of the diagnosis. These feelings often come from being confronted with a life-or-death situation (especially after a heart attack) or from having to make lifestyle changes with which they are not initially comfortable. These strong emotional responses (especially depression) can contribute to decreased sexual desire or a reduced ability to perform sexually. If you experience any of these feelings, fears, or difficulties during sexual activity, it is important to speak to a professional with whom you feel comfortable. This may be your medical doctor or a counselor specializing in sexual difficulties. During this time it is very common to have fears and anxieties related to sexual activity, so don't be embarrassed to speak up.

THE NITTY GRITTY

When can I get back to my regular life after a heart attack?

Recovering from a heart attack usually takes somewhat longer than recovering from a simple angioplasty. This is because the heart attack causes damage to the heart muscle, which is not the case during an angioplasty procedure that opens a blockage in the absence of a heart attack. If you have had a heart attack, it will likely take a bit longer to return to everyday activities. The actual length of time will depend upon a variety of factors, including the extent of the heart attack and how well you recovered while in the hospital following the heart attack. Other factors to consider are the type of treatment you are receiving and your baseline level of fitness (if you were fit prior to your heart attack, you will have a quicker recovery). As with angioplasty, your return to work will depend upon what type of a job you have. You should talk to your doctor about when it is safe for you to go back to work and return to other activities.

CHAPTER

Five

Learning to Live the
Heart♥SMART® Way

QUESTION **26** ————————

Michael is recovering well from his angioplasty and has received medical clearance to begin exercising. He has discovered that the very exercise routine that brought on the chest pain before his procedure now gives him no pain at all. He can do this exercise and more!

Since the procedure, Michael has been thinking a lot about his health and his life. Recently Jessica and he sat together on the old couch in the den and watched their favorite crime show, just as they have been doing since she was fifteen. During a commercial for life insurance, Jessica took his hand.

"Dad," she whispered, blinking away a tear, "I'm so glad we didn't have to worry about your life insurance a few weeks ago. So will you please make sure that you take care of yourself. I want you to be around for a long, long time."

Michael is thankful because he knows that at the first sign of heart disease he should have made the important life changes his doctors recommended. He is grateful that the stent has given him another chance to get it right. He is regaining his strength and healing well. Now the question at the top of his mind is . . .

I'm feeling much better. What's next for me?

THE BOTTOM LINE

Just like Michael, Diane, Rosa, Brian, and Reginald, you have been given another chance to stay alive. Now that you are recovering from your heart procedure, it is time to take charge of your health and give yourself a chance to *really* live. In fact, there is no time to lose. Your body has given you a loud, clear message. It is begging you to listen. You have the opportunity to take steps that will help you become healthier, minimize any further damage to your heart, and enjoy your life for as long as possible.

We want to help you take your first steps toward heart health. We know that it can be difficult to know exactly where to begin, so we have developed a clear, manageable five-step tool to help you launch your new, healthier lifestyle. It's called *Heart♥SMART*, and the acronym means

- **Stress reduction**
- **Medication**
- **Active lifestyle**
- **Real food**
- **Tobacco cessation**

Each of these areas is an important building block of the *Heart♥SMART* program. So, throughout this chapter and the next, we will teach you how to take steps to incorporate all of them into your new lifestyle.

It's a lot of change. I'm not sure I can do it!

It *is* true that you will have to make some significant life changes to make sure your heart disease doesn't get worse. That being said, if you try to change everything at once, it will feel overwhelming and you may not be able to sustain the changes for very long. But slow, gradual change is much more likely to produce results that you can sustain the rest of your life. As we discuss each step of the *Heart♥SMART* program, we will offer ways to help you achieve the kind of success that you can maintain in the long run.

I've never been good at staying motivated. How do I change that?

You're not alone. When it comes to making healthy changes, many people have difficulty staying motivated. The key is to find the ways that works for *you*. Motivation comes in many forms and from many places. Here are eleven ideas that have motivated some of the people with whom we've worked:

- Realize that making changes will give you more years with your partner.
- Think about being at a child's or grandchild's graduation or wedding.
- Know that for the rest of your life, poor health is much more expensive than good health.
- Make changes slowly and get used to one change before making another change.
- Look at measurable results (pounds lost, lowering your bad cholesterol number, the amount of time you are able to exercise, clearer lungs).
- Articulate goals to a friend or family member and then hold yourself responsible to that person.
- Pay a trainer, a nutritionist, or a counselor, because a financial investment will make you feel like you have to stick to your goals.
- Make healthy changes a planned part of each day's schedule, regardless of how busy you are.
- Focus on what you have already accomplished rather than the changes that still need to happen. Feel positive and optimistic about the steps you still need to take to become healthier.
- Find a friend or an organized group that is working toward the same goals and benefit from the outside support and encouragement (join a walking group or yoga class, create a healthy cooking club for a few friends).
- Write down your goals and actions each day: food eaten, minutes exercised, medications taken, etc.

My doctor suggested cardiac rehab. What is that and should I do it?

If you have had a heart attack, received a stent, or had a bypass, you are eligible to receive cardiac rehabilitation. In fact, we consider cardiac rehab to be an integral part of the *Heart♥*SMART program. By opting to take advantage of all that cardiac rehab has to offer, you will move a little closer to your health goals.

In order to begin cardiac rehab, you will need a prescription from your cardiologist. You will usually begin rehab a few weeks after your heart attack, perhaps a little sooner if you have had a stent or bypass without having had a heart attack. Cardiac rehab takes place at special rehab centers that are not typically part of a hospital but may be attached to it.

You should expect to attend rehab five days a week for about four to six weeks. Rehab will offer you several advantages.

1. You will have the opportunity to meet other people who understand all that you are experiencing because they, too, are going through the very same experiences. You may even make a new friend.
2. You will exercise with supervision until you feel confident.
3. You will learn an exercise routine that you will be able do on your own.
4. You will have opportunities to attend a variety of support groups that can help you learn how to make positive lifestyle changes in all the important areas.

THE NITTY GRITTY

There may be periods of time when you are feeling highly motivated, and you will therefore experience success at making changes toward better health. This is most likely to be during the time just after your angioplasty or heart attack, when you are confronted with a serious health issue or even with your mortality. As you begin to feel healthier, you might find that it is harder to stay motivated. This is likely because the fear of experiencing serious health issues diminishes over time.

For this reason, we suggest that you *start a journal* before the fear and motivation have faded. This journal can be any type of notebook, or you can begin journaling on your computer. It doesn't matter whether you start the journal before your angioplasty or after. Likewise, your writing style and grammatical accuracy are not important. You don't need to show your journal to anyone.

Your goal is simply to document everything you feel and experience physically and emotionally. Write about your thoughts, feelings, and experiences in as much detail as possible, including how you felt during any tests and procedures, the way this process has impacted your relationships, and what you worry about.

Journaling serves two purposes. First, many people find it very helpful to write about their feelings, especially during stressful times. But even more important, if your motivation fades as your health improves, it can be *very* useful to revisit early journal entries as a gentle reminder that if you don't continue taking the necessary steps to maintain your well-being, you could easily cause your heart health to deteriorate again and your heart disease to get worse. So start journaling *right now*!

We are now ready to discuss the *Heart♥*SMART program. For the time being, we will skip the *S* (stress). We will come back to that in chapter 6. Instead, we will begin our discussion by talking about the various medications that your doctor might prescribe. We like to start with *M* because, although every part of *Heart♥*SMART is important, taking your medication is the *most important* of the five steps. In addition, most people find this to be the easiest of the five changes to make immediately and also the least complicated to stick with in the long run.

Beginning in chapter 6, we will discuss the other four components of *Heart♥*SMART. In case you're wondering how important each of these steps is, you should know that every one is important. But if you're a smoker, the next most important step—after taking your medications—is to quit smoking. The next important step to quitting smoking is your changing your eating and exercise habits.

If you're not a smoker, these two together rank second, right behind taking medications. Reducing your stress is the least important of the steps, but don't leave it out, because, as you will see, it is definitely associated with heart health.

QUESTION 27

Each day Rosa is becoming a bit more optimistic as her health improves and she feels herself growing stronger. She is once again starting to enjoy time with her grandkids, although she's not quite ready to baby-sit. As part of her recovery, each day Rosa methodically takes the five different medications that her doctor has prescribed. She is careful to follow the directions on each bottle as well as those given to her by her cardiologist, but sometimes it is a bit overwhelming to remember which pill to take at what time. Rosa wants to do her best to follow all the medical advice, but sometimes she wonders . . .

My doctor has given me five different medications. Isn't this too much?

THE BOTTOM LINE

Even if it feels like you are taking too many medications, *it is extremely important to take **all** your medications as they were prescribed by your doctor.* Each medication has a purpose, and each one treats a different aspect of your heart health. If you aren't sure why you're supposed to be taking a particular medication, ask your doctor or pharmacist or check a reliable Internet resource for more information. Sometimes a medication can be adjusted or even discontinued. You shouldn't skip doses, however. And never stop taking a medication without first consulting your doctor.

How does my doctor decide which medications are right for me?

Actually there is a standard *cardiac cocktail* that serves as the basis for treating almost every patient diagnosed with heart disease. The cocktail is a combination of medications that, after numerous studies, have been proven to reduce the risk of future cardiovascular events (heart attack, the need for further angioplasty or bypass surgery, and even cardiac death). Each patient is prescribed a slightly different cocktail based on his or her specific risk factors as well as the specific type and level of heart disease. In addition, over time, medications will be monitored and sometimes adjusted.

The cardiac cocktail contains multiple basic medications in four classes (more about these in The Nitty Gritty), but sometimes additional medication is needed for other medical conditions. These medications address the major risk factors for CAD: high cholesterol, high blood pressure, and diabetes. In some cases, additional medication may be prescribed to help a patient quit smoking. These medications are extremely important, but like the stent procedure, they only provide a partial solution to the problem of heart health, albeit an important part. Each of these medications works best in conjunction with a healthy, balanced lifestyle (more on this in chapter 6).

Am I going to experience any side effects?

It is certainly important to understand the possible side effects of the medications that you are taking, but this doesn't mean that you will experience all or even any of them. When you read the informational insert that comes with your medications, or information about it on medical or pharmaceutical websites, you will typically find a very long list of *every* possible side effect. This extremely comprehensive list is reported for legal reasons, and it is important to remember this in order to alleviate anxiety you may feel when reading it. The best way to learn which side effects are more likely to occur is to ask your doctor. Don't rely only on your friends for this information, because while they mean well, their insights might be incorrect or may not apply to you. A friend may appear to have the same medical issues as you and may even be taking the same medications, but you can never be sure about your friend's exact diagnosis or how his or her body might be responding to a particular medication or combination of medications. It also is possible that your friend's side effect might be caused by something other than what he or she believes.

Finally, resist the urge to rely on the media for your primary education about a medication, because there is a good chance that you will receive incomplete or sensationalized information. When you educate yourself with reliable information about your medication, including benefits and side effects, you will more likely appreciate your doctor's reason for prescribing it. However, if you do experience anything with which you are not comfortable, tell your doctor, because it may be possible to change the dosage or switch the medication to something else.

What are drug interactions? Will they hurt me?

Drug interactions occur when you take two or more medications that interact with each other inside your body, causing a change in the way one or both affects your body. Drug interactions are not uncommon, but that does not necessarily mean they are bad. In fact, some drug interactions are beneficial. When combined inside your body, they may be even more effective. In general, cardiac medications are tolerated well and without problematic interactions. That said, if you take medication for medical concerns other than your heart, be sure to tell *all* your doctors about *all* your prescriptions so they can make sure there are no potentially negative or even dangerous interactions. In addition, it is a good idea to discuss all your medications with your pharmacist. Most pharmacists are very knowledgeable and well versed in potential side effects and drug interactions. We strongly recommend that you fill all your prescriptions at the same pharmacy so the pharmacist can see everything you are taking and be on the lookout for any conflicts.

THE NITTY GRITTY

Tell me more about the medications in the cardiac cocktail.

As we said above, there are four classes of medications in the basic cardiac cocktail, and each medication addresses a major risk factor for CAD.

1. Anti-platelet agents

These medications reduce the risk of heart attack. They are known as blood thinners because they prevent the blood from forming a clot that could cause a heart attack (see Question 2 for information about how a heart attack develops).

The most commonly used anti-platelet medication is aspirin (unless you are allergic to it). Aspirin is sometimes recommended for people who have risk factors for heart disease but don't yet display any of the known signs for it. Aspirin works by preventing the circulating blood platelets from sticking to one other and forming a blood clot.

If you take aspirin regularly, you might have noticed that a minor cut will bleed longer than it did before you began your aspirin regimen. This is because it takes longer to form the small clot that will stop the cut from bleeding.

Individuals with stents usually take a second blood thinner as well because, until the blood vessel heals, they are at a higher risk for forming a clot inside the stent. This is known as *dual anti-platelet therapy*. In the United States there are three anti-platelet medications available in addition to aspirin: clopidogrel (Plavix), prasugrel (Effient), and ticagrelor (Brilinta). When taking one of these drugs, you might notice that you bruise much more easily. This is not necessarily a bad thing, because it means that the medication is doing its job—thinning your blood. Most people are able to manage this minor bleeding (a bruise is actually bleeding just below the skin's surface) without a problem and are able to continue taking the medication. If you experience, however, any significant bleeding while taking one of these medications, tell your doctor right away. Never stop taking a medication without first talking to your doctor, especially if you recently had a stent procedure.

2. Cholesterol medication

Statins are the main type of medication used to lower cholesterol. You are probably familiar with the brand names of many statins because they are frequently advertised on television and through other media outlets. Statins include lovastatin (Mevacor), fluvastatin (Lescol), pravastatin (Pravachol), simvastatin (Zocor), atorvastatin (Lipitor), rosuvastatin (Crestor), and pitavastatin (Livalo). You have probably noticed that the generic name for all of these drugs ends in the suffix *statin*, hence the name. Statins all work in the same way to lower cholesterol, but they differ in terms of potency. In the list above, the weaker statins are listed in the beginning and the more potent ones toward the end.

The primary goal of the statins is to lower LDL cholesterol (the bad cholesterol); however, they actually do much more than this. They also lower C-reactive protein (CRP), which is a marker for inflammation throughout your body. Many medical professionals believe that inflammation is responsible for the development of atherosclerosis (blockages and hardening of blood vessels). When inflammation is reduced, the development of atherosclerosis is delayed or even stopped. Currently, there are no medications specifically designed to reduce inflammation, although there is ongoing research to discover a medication specifically for this purpose. For now, statins are relatively good at suppressing inflammation and reducing CRP. We will discuss statins and other cholesterol-reducing medications in greater detail in Question 28.

3. Blood pressure medication

Some people with CAD do not require medication for high blood pressure, but research reveals that more than 80 percent of individuals with CAD also have high blood pressure (hypertension) and require medication.

There are several classes (or types) of blood pressure medication. In order to control blood pressure effectively, it is not uncommon for someone to take multiple blood pressure medications, usually one from each class.

In addition to controlling blood pressure, these medications are sometimes used after a patient has had a heart attack, even when his or her blood pressure is normal. They help the heart heal more efficiently and have other beneficial effects as well. We will discuss these medications in greater detail in Question 30.

4. Diabetes medication

As you know, diabetes is a major risk factor for developing CAD, and more than one-fourth of CAD patients have diabetes and require medication. In addition, a diagnosis of diabetes complicates the treatment of CAD, and patients with diabetes tend to have less optimal outcomes. It is therefore *extremely important* to control diabetes as much as possible. If you have diabetes, your cardiologist may refer you to an endocrinologist (a doctor specializing in hormonal disorders, including diabetes) to make sure you are taking the right combination of medications to ensure the best possible results. We will discuss this in greater detail in Question 28.

QUESTION **28**

Brian is the type of person who pays close attention to details, especially when it comes to his health. He is certainly not shy about asking questions, and he goes to each medical appointment with a list of queries for his doctor. Brian now understands that one of the most important ways to avoid another heart attack is to take all the medications that are prescribed for him. He also wants to understand in detail how each medication is contributing to his overall heart health. Most of it makes sense to him, but the reason for one p rescription is puzzling him. He adds a question to the list to ask his doctor at his next appointment . . .

My cholesterol is normal. Do I really need cholesterol medication?

THE BOTTOM LINE

Yes, you do. A great deal of research has examined the benefits of long-term statin therapy.[16] This research reveals that, not only are statins extremely effective at reducing cholesterol, but they are excellent at reducing the chances of heart attack, stroke, and even death! Therefore, if you have suffered a heart attack, it is critical that you to take a statin, regardless of whether you have high cholesterol. You will be glad to know that this class of medications is extremely well tolerated by those who take it, and they have very few serious side effects. It is for these reasons that Lipitor is and has, for many years, been the best-selling medication in the world.

How exactly will I benefit from a statin if I have normal cholesterol?

This question has been evaluated in numerous clinical studies, and the research reveals that people with normal and even low cholesterol have benefits similar to patients who have elevated cholesterol.[17,18] The reason for these benefits is not completely clear, but one possible explanation is that it is due to a reduction in inflammation (see Question 2). Another possible reason that statins help everyone is that perhaps the current definition of normal cholesterol is not accurate. Current guidelines for healthy people consider a total cholesterol of 200 mg/dl and an LDL cholesterol of less than 130 mg/dl to be normal. However, we know that a normal LDL among people in rural China is less than 50 mg/dl. Not surprisingly, there is virtually no CAD in this population. In addition, the LDL goal for patients with CAD is much lower than current US guidelines. Research in this area continues, but evidence continues to mount suggesting that an LDL level of 50–70 mg/dl may be normal and optimal. This is a level achieved by almost no one in the Western world.

Can I achieve these results with diet alone?

Cholesterol comes from two major sources. The first is from your diet, and it is certainly possible to adjust your dietary intake of cholesterol by limiting or avoiding foods that contain high cholesterol levels, such as eggs, red meat, and cheese (shellfish should be limited to three cooked ounces once a week). However, even if you do this, it is not likely to result in a cholesterol level low enough to be considered optimal. This is because your liver actually produces cholesterol, and the amount of cholesterol it produces is most likely determined by your genetic makeup and is unaffected by your diet. This is why it is necessary to take a statin to properly control your cholesterol. In addition, a statin also gives you the added benefit of reducing inflammation. The bottom line is that it is important to begin a heart healthy diet (see chapter 6) *and* to reduce your liver cholesterol with a statin.

What are the side effects of statins?

Despite what you may have heard about statins (there is some very negative press about statins in the media), this class of medication is not only extremely effective but extraordinary safe. In fact, there are not very many prescription medications that are as widely used as statins and as well tolerated.

The most common side effect of statins is muscle aches or muscle weakness. This occurs in up to 5 percent of users, and it usually resolves when the medication is stopped. A very rare, more serious side effect is a muscle condition called *rhabdomyolysis*. This is the breakdown of muscle fibers, leading to the release of muscle fiber contents (myoglobin) into the bloodstream. Myoglobin is harmful to the kidneys and often causes kidney damage. Therefore, if you develop muscle aches or weakness while taking a statin, be sure to tell your doctor right away. Your doctor may instruct you to stop taking this particular statin and prescribe a different one. This is because you might have a side effect from one statin but tolerate another one with no problems.

Another potentially dangerous side effect is liver damage. This is very rare, but it might mean you will have to stop taking the statin. In most cases, there is no permanent liver damage after the medication has been discontinued. To ensure that this side effect is noticed at an early stage, your doctor will ask you to have regular blood tests.

Other rare side effects include memory loss, fatigue, lack of energy, generalized weakness, and loss of libido (sex drive). Should you experience any of these rare side effects, you will be comforted to know that all these symptoms typically resolve when the medication is stopped.

Will I see an immediate benefit?

The medication will start to work immediately, and it will only take a few weeks until your cholesterol levels fall into the target range. But even when your cholesterol reaches the right level, you won't feel any different than you did when your cholesterol was too high. Since there isn't an external change, some people believe that the medicine isn't doing anything to help them, so they stop taking it. Don't be fooled. Statins are working even when you feel no different. They can stop blockages from getting worse and prevent new blockages from forming. Since they are such an important medication for controlling CAD, be sure that you take your statin regularly and as directed.

THE NITTY GRITTY

What if the side effects make it too difficult for me to tolerate taking a statin?

It is true that a small number of people experience such extreme muscle aches or liver problems that they can no longer take a statin medication. If this happens to you, there are other medications that reduce LDL, primarily by blocking the absorption of cholesterol in the small intestine. In other words, they mimic a low cholesterol diet. Unfortunately, they do not address the cholesterol that is produced by the liver. These medications are, therefore, typically less effective than statins, and there is currently no data that demonstrates that they save lives (while there is an abundance of data to that effect for statins). For these reasons, these medications are a second line of treatment and prescribed only for those people who cannot tolerate statins or who are on the maximum statin dose but still have elevated cholesterol levels.

What do I do if my HDL (good cholesterol) is too low?

As you learned in Question 28, it is important for both your total cholesterol and your LDL to be as low as possible. In addition (*not* instead), it is also important for your HDL (protective cholesterol) to be as *high* as possible. HDL has a very important job; it is responsible for taking cholesterol (and the plaque from the cholesterol) out of the blood and transporting it to the liver. A healthy HDL is less than 35 mg/dl in men and less than 45 mg/dl in women. Fortunately for women, they typically have higher HDL than men.

It is not easy to raise your HDL, but you can raise it a moderate amount by

- Exercising regularly
- Eating a heart healthy diet (more on this in Questions 33 and 34)
- Consuming a modest amount of alcohol (one-half to one alcoholic drink a day has been show to support heart health)
- Taking a fish-oil supplement

There are medications that increase HDL, but they are much less effective than statins at decreasing LDL. In addition, they have not been proven to prevent heart attacks and save lives. The medication most commonly used to raise HDL is niacin. However, due to untoward side effects (a flushing or burning sensation and restlessness), niacin is not usually well tolerated. Large research studies are underway to evaluate medications that increase HDL dramatically; however, they are not yet FDA approved, and it is not yet clear whether they can reduce heart attacks or cardiac deaths.

How do statins work?

Total cholesterol is made up of many different particles, the two most important of these are LDL (low-density lipoprotein), which is harmful to your body, and HDL (high-density lipoprotein), which is protective. Statins reduce the level of LDL by blocking its production in the liver (but they have only minimal effects on HDL). To achieve maximum benefit from a statin, your doctor will aim to reduce your LDL to less than 100 mg/dl (or even lower) by monitoring your dosage or even switching you to a more potent statin.

Some research suggests that LDL levels below 70 mg/dl may be even more optimal in preventing the progression of CAD. In fact, some studies have shown that achieving ultralow LDL levels may lead to minor shrinking of cholesterol plaques or blockages in the arteries.

Statins may also have additional beneficial effects, unrelated to the reduction of LDL, that are not yet fully understood. Benefits not connected to LDL reduction are called *pleiotropic effects*. In addition, as we discussed, statins reduce CRP, a marker of inflammation in the body.

Researchers believe that when LDL is reduced dramatically, the pleiotropic effects are also more pronounced.

Q U E S T I O N **29** _____

Diane is home from rehab and continuing to recover. She has almost fully healed from the bypass surgery, although she still gets very tired by the end of the day. Diane realizes that her road to recovery is still quite a way off, because she needs to take important steps to become healthier. She hasn't smoked since the surgery, although she definitely worries that not smoking will be hard to stick to it. She is considering beginning a program to help her quit for good. Diane also wonders about her other risk factors. There's nothing she can do about her family history, but she wonders about everything else. At her next visit to the doctor, Diane wants to ask . . .

I have diabetes. Does this make things worse?

THE BOTTOM LINE

It might not be what you want to hear, but unfortunately, having diabetes does increase your risk for several serious medical problems. These include

- CAD, including an increased risk of heart attacks

- PAD, including an increased risk of stroke and risk of decreased blood flow to the legs
- Kidney damage, including possible kidney failure, which in some people may over time lead to the need for dialysis
- Eye damage, possibly leading to blindness
- Nerve damage

In fact, the number-one cause of diabetes-related death is CAD or PAD (including heart attack and stroke). The American Diabetes Association (ADA) reports that two out of every three people with diabetes die due to cardiovascular disease. Since these risks are so significant, the ADA recommends regular screening for early signs of damage.

If you have been diagnosed with diabetes, you are not alone. In fact, more than a quarter of people diagnosed with CAD have diabetes, and the numbers are rapidly rising. In some areas of the world (like India) the rate is as high as 50 percent. Diabetes is an epidemic in the developed world, especially in the United States. This is most likely due to lifestyle: a lack of exercise combined with the consumption of too many unhealthy foods.

Despite these facts, most people with diabetes are not aware of the connection between diabetes, heart attack, and stroke. A survey conducted in 2009 by the ADA revealed that 68 percent of people with diabetes did not feel they were at risk for cardiovascular disease, and 60 percent of diabetics surveyed did not feel that high blood pressure or cholesterol was an area of concern for them.

What exactly is diabetes?

Diabetes is a *metabolic disorder*, which means that the body is unable to properly process sugar (technically known as glucose). A large part of the food we eat is broken down into glucose, which serves as the main source of the body's energy. After food is digested, glucose enters the bloodstream through the small intestine. When your body is functioning healthily, the glucose is then moved from the bloodstream into the cells, where it is needed by a hormone called insulin. Insulin is secreted by the pancreas (a large gland behind the stomach). When a person does not have diabetes, the pancreas automatically produces the right amount of insulin needed to move the glucose from the blood into the cells.

Diabetes develops when the pancreas does not make enough insulin, when the cells in the muscles, liver, and fat do not use the insulin properly, or both. When this happens, glucose accumulates in the blood in higher-than-normal levels. There are actually two types of diabetes. Type 1 diabetes is thought to be a consequence from an autoimmune disorder and is typically diagnosed in childhood. In Type 1 diabetes, the insulin-producing cells in the pancreas do not work at all, and thus Type 1 diabetics cannot produce any insulin. Type 2 diabetes typically occurs later in life and has a genetic component (which is why it frequently runs in families), but is also connected to lifestyle. In other words, there is a genetic predisposition to develop Type 2 diabetes that is exacerbated by a sedentary lifestyle and obesity. Type 2 diabetes develops when a person does not have enough insulin to move the sugar into the cells or when the body stops being able to use the insulin correctly. The result is high levels of glucose (sugar) in the blood.

What does diabetes have to do with my heart?

The excess glucose can attach to proteins in the blood vessels and alter their normal structure and function. In addition, diabetes frequently damages the very small vessels throughout the entire body (this is known as *microcirculation*), which can lead to the vessels becoming thicker and less elastic. In the worst cases, blockages develop. Therefore diabetics often have more advanced CAD (more extensive blockages) than nondiabetics. In addition, due to nerve damage caused by the diabetes, they may have atypical symptoms or they may have no symptoms (like chest pain) that would normally serve as a warning that

CAD has developed. This is exactly why Diane had so many blockages and why she required a bypass without having any symptoms.

For all these reasons, it is more difficult to treat people with diabetes. It is harder to diagnosis them in a timely manner and more challenging to make an accurate diagnosis. In addition, it is more difficult to offer successful therapeutic options. Diabetics frequently need more extensive and more complicated procedures, a larger number of stents, or (like Diane) bypass surgery. Since diabetics require so many more interventions, their risk for complications during procedures is also higher. What's more, diabetics are more likely to have stent re-blockages (restenosis) and bypasses that become blocked more quickly. This is especially true among diabetics who require insulin therapy.

What can I do to reduce my risk?

You will be comforted to know that diabetes can be controlled by reversing an unhealthy lifestyle. Regular exercise, weight loss, and a healthy eating program can dramatically improve blood sugar levels and in some cases even result in a reversal of the diagnosis. If you are able to eliminate your diabetes or even control it, this will have a dramatic and positive impact on preventing your CAD from getting worse. Controlling your diabetes will also help significantly to keep stents and bypasses open and reduce the risk for future heart attacks and stroke.

If you require medication to control diabetes, it is important that you begin treatment immediately. The sooner you are able to control your blood sugar levels, the quicker and more effectively you will reduce your risk of cardiovascular complications. However, please remember that the medication is *much more effective* when used in conjunction with exercise and a healthy diet. Medication is not a substitute for these. You will have a much better chance of long-term success and you may require less medication if you focus on adopting a healthy lifestyle (more on this in chapter 6).

THE NITTY GRITTY

How will I know whether my diabetes is controlled?

There are two ways to determine whether diabetes is under control. The first is to check your blood sugar level by pricking your finger and extracting a small amount of blood to test with a personal monitor. This is typically accomplished when you wake up in the morning (in order to get a fasting glucose level). If you take insulin, you may be instructed to check your blood at other times during the day in order to determine how much insulin you need.

The other way to see whether your diabetes is controlled is for your doctor to take a blood sample for a hemoglobin A1c test. This test reflects your average blood sugar level over the prior three months. It measures the amount of sugar that is attached to hemoglobin (a protein in red blood cells). Hemoglobin circulates in the blood for about three months, so by looking at the amount of sugar attached to the hemoglobin, your doctor is able to make a fairly good assessment as to how much sugar has also bound to other proteins. This assessment is an indication of your overall blood sugar level for that period of time. If the hemoglobin carries a lot of glucose, it means that there is a good chance that proteins in your blood vessels do too, which can cause them to become damaged. On the other hand, if the hemoglobin A1c test reveals that the hemoglobin is not bound with very much sugar, it means that you have good blood sugar control and a lower risk of tissue damage.

If you have diabetes, you should have your hemoglobin screened several times a year to make sure that your treatment plan is working. This will help you determine if your diet program and exercise routine are satisfactory, and it will also help your doctor evaluate how you are responding to medications. A normal hemoglobin A1c level is less than or equal to 5.9 percent, but for diabetics, a level of about 7 percent indicates adequate control of blood sugar levels. It is not advisable for diabetics to lower their hemoglobin A1c to a near normal level, because this can cause complications related to blood sugar levels being too low. In clinical studies, hemoglobin A1c that is too low has not been shown to be beneficial and can even be harmful.[19] However, levels above 8 percent indicate poor control of diabetes and should be addressed as soon as possible.

Are there any other medical issues about which I, as a diabetic, should be concerned?

As we have discussed, having diabetes is a risk factor for developing CAD. In addition, being overweight (also a risk factor for CAD) can lead to Type 2 diabetes. *Central obesity* (which is when you carry extra weight around your waist rather than your hips) is most closely associated with developing diabetes. A waist measurement of more than forty inches for men or thirty-five inches for women indicates central obesity. Central obesity also raises your risk for heart disease, because abdominal fat can increase the production of LDL cholesterol (bad cholesterol), which can deposit blood fat onto the blood vessel walls. In addition, those with central obesity who are also diabetic frequently have elevated triglyceride levels. Triglycerides are a different form of blood fat that increases your risk for CAD. To complicate matters even further, many diabetics have low levels of HDL (good cholesterol), which protects them from CAD.

In addition to weight and cholesterol issues, diabetics have almost double the risk for developing high blood pressure (hypertension) than those who are not diabetic. As you can see, it is important to do your best to keep your diabetes in control as it is so closely associated with several other CAD risk factors. The better you are able to control these risk factors, the more likely you are to reduce your risk for further CAD.

What can I do about this?

Being diagnosed with diabetes does not mean that a heart attack or stroke is inevitable. To reduce your risk of suffering either of these, health care professionals recommend that diabetics engage in a comprehensive treatment plan in order to reduce the risk of CAD. The plan asks diabetics to watch their ABCs. In this case:

A is for [hemoglobin] A1c: This blood test is considered the best way to measure glucose levels, and so diabetics are recommended to be tested at least twice a year.

B is for blood pressure (hypertension): Hypertension, a risk factor for CAD, can only be controlled if it is recognized. Diabetics should aim to achieve a blood pressure below 130/80 mmHg. In Question 30 we will discuss hypertension in greater detail.

C is for cholesterol: Ideally, LDL cholesterol levels should be below 100 mg/dl and HDL levels should be greater than 40 mg/dl for men and 50 mg/dl for women. A healthy diet, regular exercise, weight loss, and medication should all be part of your plan to achieve your cholesterol goals.

QUESTION 30

When Reginald first learned that he was not a candidate for an angioplasty, he was secretly disappointed. He had hoped that he would be able to get a stent and then go back to his regular life (except for the fights with his wife). Instead, Reginald's cardiologist explained that he has many blockages, but none of them are severe enough to warrant angioplasty. By adopting a healthier lifestyle and taking his medications as prescribed, Reginald should be able to slow or stop the progression of the blockages. He told Reginald that healthier eating, exercise, and medications would be his recommendation, even if Reginald did require a stent. *When Reginald realized that a stent is not a quick fix, he stopped feeling disappointed. Instead, he began to focus on his medications. Reginald has never been the kind of person to take medications, so now he does not want to take any more than absolutely necessary. When contemplating the bottle of blood pressure pills, Reginald thinks that maybe he can do without these. He immediately calls his doctor's office to ask . . .*

My blood pressure is high, but I feel fine.
Can I manage it without medication?

THE BOTTOM LINE

As we discussed in Question 29, high blood pressure (hypertension) is one of the major risk factors for heart attacks and strokes. Normal blood pressure is at or below 120/80 mmHg. This is normally measured at rest and should be confirmed on at least two different occasions. You will know that you have hypertension if your systolic blood pressure (the top number on the reading) is above 140 mmHg or if your diastolic pressure (the bottom number) is above 90 mmHg. Aside from these measurements, there is a good chance that you will not know whether you have high blood pressure. Unless their blood pressure is extremely high, most people (like Reginald) feel absolutely fine, with no symptoms at all. It is therefore possible to have hypertension for many years before being diagnosed. It is even possible for your first symptom to be a heart attack or stroke! Therefore, notwithstanding how you feel, it is very important for everyone to check his or her blood pressure on a regular basis. Your primary care physician or cardiologist can do this for you, or you can even do it yourself at a pharmacy or fire station.

Why is hypertension bad?

High blood pressure damages your blood vessels (arteries) because the higher pressure forces the vessels to endure greater stress than is desired. This stress can lead to a loss of *arterial elasticity*, which means that the arteries will become stiffer and can eventually develop blockages.

As we noted earlier, the heart is a muscle. When it is forced to work harder than normal—pumping against high blood pressure—the work will lead to a thickening of the muscle. In most other instances, building muscle is a desirable outcome, because it increases strength and bone density. However, building heart muscle is not a positive result, and it can lead to a number of different problems, like congestive heart failure. In addition, your brain does not tolerate high blood pressure well at all, which is why hypertension increases the risk of stroke.

Do I have to take medication if I have hypertension?

If you are diagnosed with hypertension, you may need medication, but the optimal treatment for you will depend upon the severity of your hypertension. It is important to do everything possible to reduce your blood pressure, because reduction of the systolic blood pressure by only 5 mmHg can decrease the risk of stroke by 34 percent and reduce your chances of CAD by 21 percent.[20]

It is possible that, before trying medication, your doctor will suggest that you first try several lifestyle changes. These are proven to control blood pressure in many cases and may allow you to avoid the need for medication.

1. **Regular exercise can relieve hypertension.** You should aim for twenty to thirty minutes, five days a week, of moderate to fast-paced aerobic (cardio) exercise. Ideas for aerobic exercise

include walking, swimming, biking, and using a cross-trainer. (See chapter 6).

2. If you are overweight, **losing weight can lower your blood pressure.** (See chapter 6.)

3. A high sodium (salt) diet will increase blood pressure, because salt retains water. By slightly increasing your circulating blood volume, your blood pressure goes up. It is, therefore, important to **reduce your salt intake as much as possible.** Do not use table salt (one teaspoon contains 2.3 grams or 2,325 milligrams) and start paying attention to the nutritional information of the foods you eat. Many commercially prepared foods contain a great deal of sodium, so *read the labels on all products and aim for no more than 2 grams (or 2,000 mg) of sodium intake per day.* On those occasions that you consume too much sodium, you may notice a spike in your blood pressure.

4. Alcohol significantly raises blood pressure, so stick to the limit of **no more than one drink a day**.

5. If you are a smoker, **quit smoking.** In addition to all the other benefits of not smoking, it will make your hypertension much easier to control.

When you address all of these factors, you will find them to be a very effective basis for controlling blood pressure. That being said, you may still require medication. Keep in mind that, as with all the medications we have discussed, medication for hypertension will be *much more effective* when used in conjunction with the five life-style changes listed above. In addition, if you have CAD, have had a prior stroke, or if your blood pressure is very high, your doctor may choose to start you on medication immediately. This is because it is likely that lifestyle changes alone will not achieve the desired blood pressure goal, which is less than 130/80 mmHg in patients with CAD or diabetes; for those without these diseases, the goal is less than 140/90 mmHg.

THE NITTY GRITTY

How do I understand these numbers?

If your doctor tells you that you have high blood pressure, you can refer to the following chart to understand how high it actually is compared to a healthy blood pressure.

	Systolic BP in mmHg (the top number)	Diastolic BP in mmHg (the bottom number)
Normal	90–119	60–79
Prehypertension	120–139	80–89
Stage 1 hypertension	140–159	90–99
Stage 2 hypertension	≥160	≥100

Hypertension classification based on JNC7 [21].

What medications will be prescribed for my hypertension?

In the United States there are more than one hundred different blood pressure medications available (plus combinations of medications). The correct medication for you will depend on what medical concerns you may have in addition to hypertension. This is because many antihypertensive medications (medications to treat hypertension) have beneficial effects in addition to treating blood pressure. Therefore, when possible, your doctor will choose a medication that can address more than one medical concern. It is also possible that you will require multiple medications, because it is the combination that helps you achieve your recommended blood pressure goal.

There are several classes (types) of mediations used to treat high blood pressure. These include

- Angiotensin-converting enzyme (ACE) inhibitors
- Angiotensin II receptor blockers (ARBs)
- Diuretics
- Beta-blockers

- Calcium channel blockers
- Alpha-blockers
- Alpha-agonists
- Direct Renin inhibitors
- Combination medications

You should resist the urge to compare your medications to those of others, because doctors can vary in their recommendations.

Why am I on blood pressure medication when my blood pressure is normal?

Many individuals with CAD (especially those who have had a heart attack) take two classes of antihypertensive medications, beta-blockers, and ACE inhibitors. While people with CAD typically have hypertension, there are some that may be on these medications despite having normal blood pressure. This is because, as mentioned previously, these medications treat other diseases in addition to high blood pressure.

Beta-blockers, for example, slow the heart rate and are cardio-protective for people who have had a heart attack and for those who have had congestive heart failure. They prevent life-threatening arrhythmias, so if you fall into one of these categories, you may be advised to take a beta-blocker, even if you have low blood pressure. Similarly, when someone suffers congestive heart failure or has had a heart attack, ACE-inhibitors have been shown to prolong life. In fact, they are considered *optimal medical therapy* for these patients. For those with kidney disease or diabetes, ACE-inhibitors also protect kidneys from further damage. Those who do not tolerate ACE-inhibitors or are allergic to them can use Angiotensin II receptor blockers (ARBs), which are very similar medications and have fundamentally the same benefits.

CHAPTER

Six

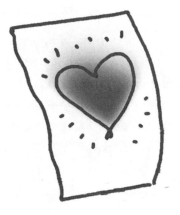

You Are Worth It!

QUESTION **31** _____

Since his heart attack, Brian has been trying to learn as much as possible about how he can stop his CAD from progressing any further. He wants to make sure he does not have another heart attack. Brian has read several articles that discuss the importance of stress reduction as an important part of heart health. Brian now realizes that his life is very stressful. In particular, his job is highly pressured with many deadlines. He also worries about his youngest son, Jeremy, who has struggled academically, but now, as a senior in high school, is threatening to quit school before graduation. Brian is also a perfectionist and a worrier. He knows that there are situations during which he feels stress that do not necessarily cause other people to feel the same way.

Brian recognizes the need to reduce the stress in his life, but he is not sure that doing so is really possible. He wonders if this will really make a difference and continues to research this question, wondering . . .

My life is stressful, but how does this affect my heart and what should I do about it?

THE BOTTOM LINE

How do I know whether I am in a stressful situation?

A great deal of research has found a strong relationship between heart disease and stress. To begin with, it is useful to know that there are two types of stressors (the event that causes you to feel stress):

- An *acute stressor* can be defined as short-term, sudden, surprising, or abrupt. Examples include the death of a loved one, losing your job, or experiencing a traumatic experience such as a robbery or a fire. A study showed that grief over the death of a significant person was associated with an acutely increased risk of a heart attack in the days following the death.[22] The risk was greatest on the first day, with a more than twentyfold increase in risk, and then declined over the next few days. The impact was greatest among individuals at high cardiovascular risk.

- A *chronic stressor* is experienced as long-term and seemingly never ending, like financial difficulties or a long-term illness of oneself or a loved one. For example, a Duke University study found that in the six months following the stock market crash of October 2008, there was a significant increase in the rate of heart attacks.[23] As another example, after Hurricane Katrina, Tulane University researchers found that the prolonged disaster—including loss of employment and health insurance and decreased access to health services—was associated with a threefold increase in heart attacks for up to two years after the hurricane.[24] Similar statistics were also evident after the Niigata-Chuetsu earthquake in Japan.[25]

While stressors (the situation that causes you to feel stress) are most often negative, they can also be positive. For example, acute stressors, like a surprise party or an exciting sporting event, are fun but might still be experienced by your body as stressful. This is also true for some chronic situations like a job promotion or a large home renovation.

In addition, stress is subjective. What you may find stressful, someone else might not. For example, while one person might find it relaxing to retire from work, someone else might find retirement to be a highly stressful transition. Everyone's ability to cope with stress is different, and it is important to understand which situations are stressful for you and how to manage them in the best way possible.

It is also important to keep in mind that for those people not at risk for CAD, stressors do not cause heart attacks. If you don't have CAD, you will not have a heart attack when a hurricane hits or you experience a personal crisis. However, people with *preexisting* CAD may be at higher risk for a heart attack when confronted with a stressor. It is important to learn your personal risk for this, because, as we have discussed, most people do not know that they have or are at risk for developing CAD.

How do I know if I am stressed?

There are many different signs that indicate you may be experiencing stress. For example, the emotions associated with stress are negative. These include

- Anxiety, worrying
- Anger
- Frustration
- Helplessness
- Feeling overwhelmed
- Confusion
- Distracted, difficulty concentrating
- Depression, sadness, crying

Stress can also cause physical symptoms such as

- Headache
- Stomachache
- Dizziness
- Heart palpitations

How does stress trigger a heart attack?

The medical community is not completely sure how stress triggers a heart attack for those with CAD. The most likely reason is that very high stress levels cause certain hormonal changes that can lead to a plaque rupture at the site of an existing blockage. This sudden rupture of plaque and subsequent attachment to the vessels of a blood clot can lead to a sudden full blockage, causing a heart attack. The stress hormone cortisol is also thought to be associated with heart attack risk. Researchers in Israel found higher concentrations of hair cortisol in patients who suffered heart attacks [26] compared with a control population. This research suggests that chronic stress (assessed by the increased levels of cortisol) in the three months prior to the heart attack may be a contributing factor for heart attacks.

Another clue that heart attacks are associated with stress comes from observing when heart attacks tend to occur. Research finds that heart attacks are more likely to occur in the early morning hours, which are associated with the stress of going to work or beginning a very busy day. In addition, findings reveal that the rate of heart attacks peaks on the first day of the workweek (Monday) and then gradually declines as the week continues. One study found that when a national holiday fell on a Monday, the rate of heart attacks for that day was similar to weekend rates (low). This study also found that heart attacks occurred at a significantly higher rate on workdays than on weekends.[27] It is possible that *anticipatory anxiety* is one of the reasons that heart attacks are more likely to occur when individuals are anticipating a busy day or a busy week. A recent study among men with a mean age of sixty showed that, for older men, having an anxious personality increased the risk for having heart attacks by 43 percent.[28]

How do I reduce my stress?

Now that you understand the relationship between heart disease and stress, the next important step is to learn how to manage your stress levels so that you reduce or eliminate stress as a risk factor for having a heart attack (or another one). Remember, coping with stress is an important part of your treatment plan, so the following six steps will help you to get started.

STEP 1: Talk it out. Talking is one of the best ways to manage stress, because it allows you to share the burden with someone else and, if necessary, receive support and advice for how to manage your situation. You might want to talk to the family member with whom you feel closest. However, if you don't feel comfortable burdening your family, or if you don't want to share your feelings in this way, you can seek out a friend or even a professional, such as a therapist or counselor.

STEP 2: Sweat it out. We know that regular exercise is an important part of managing heart disease. However, it is also a very effective way to cope with stress. Moderate to heavy physical activity helps distract you for a while, lowers cortisol and other stress hormones, gives you a feeling of control over at least one part of your life, and channels your negative feelings. It's a win-win!

STEP 3: Take a deep breath. Slow, controlled breathing is a simple yet effective way to reduce the feeling of stress as it creeps up on you. Deep breathing is not like regular breathing, and it is helpful to practice it once or twice a day even when you are not feeling stressed. You will then be more likely to use it when you do need it (like when you're sitting in traffic, about to have an argument, walk in and discover a sink full of dishes, or when dinner accidentally burns).

Try it now. Place your hand on your stomach. Then breathe in for a slow count of five. As you breathe in, feel the breath move through your lungs and into your stomach, causing your stomach to expand like a balloon. Then breathe out for a slow count of five. As you breathe out, your stomach deflates. That's one deep breath. Try two to four more for a full count of three to five breaths. Try deep breathing each time you are confronted with feelings of stress.

STEP 4: Rethink your priorities. Stress is frequently caused by placing too much emphasis on situations that are not as important as they may appear. You are at a crossroads in your life. A diagnosis of heart disease or a heart attack is an opportunity to rethink what is really important to you. You will reduce your stress if you do the following:

- Forgive minor infractions (your own and those of other people) and then forget them.
- Distance yourself from relationships that are not fun or are unpleasant. Focus on relationships that are supportive and positive.
- Pick and choose your battles with others.
- Assess which aspects of your daily life cause you the most stress and try to adjust these. For example, some people find housework very stressful, but others find a messy house even more stress provoking. Ask for help to manage the areas that cause you the most stress.

STEP 5: Say "no" more than "yes." Many people experience stress because they take on more than they can reasonably accomplish. What feels manageable to one person may be stressful for another one. So don't compare yourself to others. Instead, do your best to make sure that you can accomplish your goals without feeling too rushed, too tired, or too overwhelmed. Don't take on more than you can reasonably accomplish, and resist feeling pressured to help others or do favors if it might jeopardize your own health. If this is a change for you, then you need to explain this shift to your kids, friends, and other family members and ask for their support.

STEP 6: Meditate for a moment. Learning how to meditate is a wonderful way to reduce stress levels. The positive impact of a few minutes of meditation can last several hours. There are several types of meditation, and it might sound complicated, but it is actually simple to learn. It is more complicated to do it well!

To begin, plan to meditate for five minutes. You can increase the amount of time by a minute each time as you get better at it.

1. Pick a time of day that allows you to devote the required time to meditation.

2. Choose a quiet place away from a television, phone, or any other distractions.

3. If you feel anxious about your time limit, set an alarm to ring at the end of the five minutes so you don't have to worry about whether you have meditated for too long or not long enough.

4. Sit in a comfortable position. Many people find it easiest to sit in a chair.

5. Relax your body. Take a deep breath. Clear your mind.

6. Breathe slowly, focus only on your breathing.

7. Each time you find your thoughts drifting to obligations, daily activities, or worries, refocus on your breathing. At first you might find it hard to focus on "nothing" for more than a couple of seconds.

8. Meditate every day. Each time, try to focus on your breathing for a bit longer. Eventually you should be able to focus for the full five minutes. When the meditation becomes easier, add a bit more time.

THE NITTY GRITTY

I heard that watching football can cause a heart attack. Is that true?

Unfortunately, in some cases it is true. For some people, watching sporting events can increase their risk of heart attack and death. The rates are highest for those with CAD and when the sports event includes one or more of the following:

- A passionate fan
- A high-stakes game
- A high-intensity game
- A loss
- A loss played at home

In such situations, anxiety, anger, and passionate feelings often precipitate heart attacks and cardiovascular death. These feelings trigger a cascade of physiological responses that cause your body to respond as if it was in a highly stressful or emergency situation. Drinking alcohol or smoking during the sporting event will make it even more difficult for your body to cope. The perceived emergency causes your heart to pump faster, thereby increasing the amount of oxygen that your heart muscle needs. At the same time, you experience a decrease in oxygen supply, an increase in the risk of arrhythmias (irregular heartbeat), and an increase in the risk of thrombosis (blood clots).

Taking beta-blockers and aspirin, practicing stress management techniques, and avoiding high-risk activities (drinking alcohol, smoking, abusing drugs or medications, eating fatty foods, and over-eating) can be helpful in reducing your risk.

What is broken-heart syndrome?

Broken-heart syndrome (also known as Takotsubo cardiomyopathy) mimics a heart attack. It has the same symptoms and clinical presentation. However, it is not actually caused by the blockage of a coronary artery. Broken-heart syndrome is characterized by a ballooning of the bottom part of the heart (called the *apex*), because that part of the heart temporarily stops working properly. The word *takotsubo* is Japanese and means "fishing pot for trapping octopus." The syndrome bears this name because when the bottom of the heart muscle is not contracting (squeezing) properly, the shape of the heart resembles a fishing pot. This is usually triggered by a sudden and intensely traumatic event or by severe stress. It is thought that elevated stress hormone levels (like adrenaline) have a negative effect on the heart, triggering the syndrome. Under most circumstances, the heart recovers completely as soon as the stressor is removed.

QUESTION **32**

A month has passed since Rosa's heart attack and she received a stent. She continues to waver between feeling worried that it could happen again and thankful that she is doing so well. At this point, Rosa's biggest goal is to begin taking care of her grandchildren again. But while she is eager to baby-sit her grandchildren, she is worried that she might have a medical crisis while she is with them. Rosa realizes that it would be a good idea to begin exercising as a way to strengthen her heart and the rest of her body. She is a bit embarrassed to admit that she has never formally exercised at any time in her life. Where to begin? Before anything else, Rosa realizes that she must ask her doctor . . .

Is it okay to be active after my heart procedure?

THE BOTTOM LINE

Yes, you can and you *should!* Once you have healed from the procedure (and heart attack, if you had one) and your doctor clears you to return to your regular activities (see Question 25), it is important to be as active as possible. In fact, in 2007 the American College of Sports Medicine (ACSM) and the American Heart Association (AHA) updated the 1995 recommendations regarding physical activity for adults.[29] Despite these physical-activity recommendations, physical inactivity remains a pressing public health concern. In 2005, for example, nearly 25 percent of adults aged eighteen to sixty-five years old reported no leisure-time activity, and less than half of US adults met the physical activity guidelines.

For people who have heart disease, there are several important physical and emotional benefits associated with regular exercise. To begin, exercise improves your cardiovascular health (heart strength) and reduces the risk of developing heart disease (or worsening it). Regular exercise also helps you to control your weight, blood pressure, and cholesterol—important risk factors for heart disease. Exercise strengthens bones, improves muscle strength, and increases balance and flexibility. Physical activity also improves your circulation, helps your body use oxygen more efficiently, and improves endurance and energy levels. Exercise can also support you emotionally. It helps to improve sleep, manage stress, and alleviate some aspects of anxiety and depression. Exercise can even improve your sex life. It strengthens your muscles and bones and can reduce your risk for developing chronic diseases that are associated with aging, which will help you live healthily for longer. The American Heart Association estimates that for *every hour* of regular exercise, you gain approximately *two hours* of additional life expectancy! We hope that by now you're convinced that exercise should be an important part of your life. That being said, before you begin to exercise, **check with your doctor** to make sure that you are healthy enough to begin an exercise program.

How do I get started?

When you have the conversation with your doctor about exercising, be sure to ask questions about the specific ways in which you can and should exercise, if there is any exercise you should avoid, and how intense your exercise program should be.

Your doctor may recommend that you begin your exercise regimen by enrolling in a cardiac rehabilitation program (see more about cardiac rehab in Question 26). You will enjoy the important benefit of professional supervision (typically by an exercise physiologist) as you begin to exercise for the first time after your procedure. This is especially important if you do not have a history of regular exercise.

You will learn which exercises you should and should not do, and you will receive support in determining how your body is tolerating the exercise.

Whether you start exercise with supervision or on your own, it is very important for you to be aware of how your body is responding to the exercise. Exercising the right way is so important that we consulted Steve Panzik, a licensed physical therapist and exercise physiologist, so that we could give you the best advice about exercising after being diagnosed with CAD.

Steve's first advice is that you need to learn to listen to your body to determine whether you are exercising correctly or too hard. Steve explains that No Pain, No Gain is *not* a good rule to follow if you feel pain, discomfort, or other unusual or abnormal signs or symptoms before, during, or after you exert yourself. If you experience any of these, tell your doctor immediately. In particular, be on the lookout for chest pain, labored (heavy) breathing, or extreme fatigue. If your symptoms do not resolve within a few minutes, call 911 immediately. This is the fastest and safest way to get immediate medical care in the event that you are having a heart attack (see Question 1).

What exactly does "regular exercise" mean?

The American Heart Association recommends at least 150 minutes per week of moderate exercise or 75 minutes of vigorous exercise (or a combination of moderate and vigorous exercise).

It is beneficial to exercise on as many days of the week as possible, leaving one to two days for rest. For example, you might want to aim for thirty minutes a day on five days a week or twenty-five minutes a day for six days a week. That being said, as you heal from surgery, Steve explains that just as Rome was not built in a day, you should not aim to return to or achieve an ideal fitness level in your first workout. It can and should take much longer. Therefore, start small and gradually build up. You can even do two or more smaller workouts within the same day rather than one long one. Keeping busy with the daily activities of life (such as household chores or shopping) is not the same as exercising, so it does not count toward your daily exercise goal. However, keeping busy rather than spending most of your time sitting *is* very important, so throughout your daily life, you should be as active as possible in addition to doing your best to achieve your exercise goals.

What type of exercise should I do?

Exercise (physical activity) can be any activity that gets you to move your body and burn calories. There are three main types of exercise: aerobic (cardio) exercise, strength training, and stretching. Aerobic exercise includes activities such as walking, jogging, biking, swimming, or using machines such as a treadmill, elliptical cross-trainer, stationary bike, or rowing machine. Of the three types, aerobic exercise offers the greatest benefit to your heart. Strength training includes exercises that strengthen your muscles, such as lifting weights and using resistance rubber bands. Stretching is just what it sounds like: activities that gently stretch the large muscles to help you become and remain flexible, which is important as we age. Steve suggests that you even try an exercise program you have never done before. For example, you may enjoy a yoga, Pilates, or tai chi class. These are all exercise routines that help you develop great overall flexibility, teaching you to stretch and move your body safely under the eyes of a professional. Before beginning your exercise program, you should ask local studios or gyms if they have a medical professional on staff who is familiar with cardiovascular disease and who can help guide you through an exercise program.

What's the best way to get started?

The first and simplest step you can take to improve your heart health is to literally take a step! Begin walking. Walking is not complicated. You already know how to do it. It can be social (if you walk with a partner) or it can be a time to catch up on an audio-book or to listen to music. When you begin a walking program, research shows that its ease and flexibility mean that you have a good chance of sticking with it and making it a regular part of your life. Another great benefit of walking is that it improves bone density, which helps prevent and fight osteoporosis. In addition, walking is low impact, so it produces less stress on your knees than does jogging or running. If you have tried walking and still feel discomfort in your knees, try walking on a treadmill or at your local track. Both of these will be easier on your knees than walking on pavement. Tracks are typically made of rubber, which decreases the shock felt through your knees.

Of course, you don't have to choose walking. In order for you to feel successful and to stick with an exercise regimen, you need to choose an activity that you enjoy that will also get your heart pumping. A stationary bike, elliptical trainer, or rowing machine is a great cardiovascular tool that causes less stress on your knees. All are fairly simple to use after you have received the proper orientation from a fitness professional.

What if I can't exercise for the full thirty minutes?

When you first start an exercise program, you should not necessarily expect to be able to do a full 30 minutes a day or even the complete 150 minutes a week. This is especially true if you did not exercise regularly (or at all) before your procedure (or heart attack). Steve strongly suggests that you keep it simple and take very small steps, even if this is only 5 minutes on a treadmill at a slow pace a couple of times a week. He explains that your goal is to gradually build up your fitness and heart strength, but he reminds us that everyone improves at a different rate, so listen to *your* body. However much you are able to accomplish is *always* better than no exercise at all! Over a period of weeks or months you can gradually increase the amount of time that you exercise. This is not an all-or-nothing accomplishment. If you think about it as a process (like building a house) and expect it to take time, you won't feel discouraged if you can't immediately do the full 30 minutes or 150 minutes.

Once you have built up your stamina, it is a good idea to include some muscle-strengthening exercises in your routine. Do not begin strength training without supervision, as excessive strain can be detrimental to your heart. It is always better to train with lighter weights and do more repetitions than to push yourself to lift too much weight. You should aim to strengthen your major muscle groups: your chest, shoulders, abdomen, back, hips, and legs. You can aim to exercise each muscle group at least twice a week, with at least forty-eight hours between exercise sessions. Strength-training exercises include lifting weights, using resistance bands, or doing exercises that use your body weight as resistance. If you are new to strength training, work with an exercise specialist to learn effective exercises and correct techniques. Remember, if you are considering working with weights, it is absolutely critical not to overdo it!

Above all, no matter what exercise you choose, take it slow. "Remember," Steve encourages, "you don't put the roof on the house until you have a solid foundation. It is important that you—with the help of your fitness professional—build that solid foundation."

This all sounds great, but how do I stay motivated?

Lack of motivation has thwarted the best intentions of many, many people who begin an exercise program. Therefore, developing strategies for staying motivated is a very important component of your new, healthy lifestyle. We would like to offer you six tips that are sure to keep you moving forward.

1. **Set concrete short-term goals.** For example, commit to exercising for ten minutes every Tuesday and Saturday for the first two weeks, then add a third day for the next two weeks. During weeks five and six, increase your time to twelve minutes at each workout. In a log, write down these short-term goals, your

accomplishments at each exercise session. For now, don't focus on the long-term goal. You will achieve a little more each time with manageable, realistic, short-term goals that aren't overwhelming. Steve suggests that you set one goal that you plan to achieve each week and a slightly longer one to achieve at the end of the month. As you progress, your goals will become a little more challenging. For example, during the first month, give yourself a goal to exercise three times each week for at least ten minutes. Your monthly goal is then twelve days of exercise.

2. **Reward yourself.** When you reach your monthly goal, reward yourself with something that you enjoy (not food!). Some examples of rewards include a movie that you want to see, a new outfit, a pedicure, or a trip to see your grandchildren.

3. **Break it up.** You will benefit from exercising even if you divide your workout time into two or three segments throughout the day. For example, to achieve your goal of thirty minutes, you might choose to take a ten-minute walk in the morning, ride a stationary bike for ten minutes in the afternoon, and take another ten-minute walk in the evening. If your initial goal is ten minutes of exercise a day, you can take a five-minute walk in the morning and another one later in the day.

4. **Keep it interesting.** Steve explains that you would not sit through a movie that you don't find interesting and you don't finish reading a book that you don't enjoy. Exercise is no different. Make your fitness fun and don't let it get boring. For example, you might take one walk a week around the mall (but not shopping!) and another around a nearby park or lake. Changing the scenery stimulates your senses and increases the likelihood that you will continue the activity. Some people prefer to stick to one type of exercise, while others enjoy a variety of physical activities so they don't get bored. A benefit to variety is that you have less chance of a muscle or ligament injury caused by the repetitive use of a particular body part.

5. **Carry a motivator.** Of course you are exercising for your own health. However, it can be very helpful to carry a picture or memento that will remind you how important it is to be healthy. For example, choose a picture of your child, grandchild, partner, or pet to keep in your pocket. On days that you lack the motivation to exercise, take a look at your picture and think about how important it is to you to continue to have time with your loved ones. Remember that this is another reason that you exercise!

6. **Calendar it.** As you can see, it is important to make exercise a part of your regular daily activity. To make sure that you achieve this, you will need to put exercise on your schedule. For example, include exercise in your morning routine right after breakfast or add an evening walk after dinner. If exercise is on your calendar, you will be more likely to stick to it. In the beginning, try exercising at different times to determine what works best for you.

THE NITTY GRITTY

Am I too old for a gym?

You are never too old to try the gym! In fact, most people enter a gym for the first time as adults. If you are nervous, try going in the early afternoon when most gyms are quiet. They are typically crowded early in the morning and after work.

When your cardiovascular rehab instructor suggests that you have progressed enough to use a gym, ask him or her to talk to a fitness professional at the gym about your fitness program. Many gyms have instructors who work specifically with individuals who have heart disease or have had a heart procedure or heart surgery. It is your job to connect your cardiovascular rehab instructor with the correct trainer at the gym. Once you do this, they can and should work together to ensure your best fitness outcome.

Should I get a trainer?

A fitness professional offers great guidance to ensure that you are on a safe path to fitness success, but you don't need a trainer every time you work out. You can engage a trainer once a week and exercise on your own the other days. Every two to four weeks you should ask the trainer to develop a new, slightly more challenging program for you so that you can continue to make progress. Make sure you feel comfortable with the trainer you choose and that he or she is knowledgeable about your medical needs. Don't keep any secrets from your trainer, because understanding your medical background allows the fitness professional to develop a safe, effective program for you. If, for any reason, you don't feel comfortable with the trainer with whom you begin, it's important to switch. Your concern should have nothing to do with the trainer's feelings, but rather you need to find someone with whom you feel comfortable and productive.

Is my balance going?

As we age it is common to gradually lose our natural sense of balance. An effective fitness program can accommodate your different systems of balance in order to decrease the risk of falls. You should speak to your cardiovascular rehab instructor or fitness trainer about this aspect of exercising. Feeling better about your balance will allow you to feel more confident in your exercise program as well as in your daily activities.

Am I too old to get stronger?

The good news is that you can improve flexibility as well as gain muscle and strength at any age! In fact, your muscles atrophy only when you don't use them. Steve explains that "if you don't use it, you lose it" definitely is true when it comes to fitness. Therefore, you should continue to use your body fully and challenge yourself safely throughout your life. It's never too late!

33

At Diane's two-week visit to her cardiologist following her bypass surgery, the doctor told Diane that she was healing right on schedule. She then explained that, in order to reduce the possibility of Diane's heart disease worsening, it was time for Diane to begin giving serious attention to her health. As she listened to the doctor, Diane felt a little overwhelmed.

"I do my best to limit how many cookies, cake, and ice cream I eat," she explained to the doctor. "I know that's important for my diabetes."

"Actually, that's not quite enough," the doctor replied. "There are a few more things that you should do to improve your heart health."

Diane left the doctor's office feeling a bit down. As soon as she got home, she called her best friend Evelyn, hoping that Evelyn would be able to help her with her biggest concern . . .

My doctor told me to eat healthily. How do I do that?

THE BOTTOM LINE

This question and Question 34 address the R component of the *Heart♥SMART* program: *real food*. It is very important to learn how to incorporate heart healthy eating into your life following your procedure or heart attack. For the most part, this means eating real, whole foods rather than processed foods. Before we begin discussing the particulars, keep in mind that this is not meant to be a diet that you will try for a few weeks and then stop. Your goal is to make a long-term change in your eating habits that you will maintain for the *rest* of your life. In order to achieve permanent change, you will need to make realistic, slow changes. Many popular very low fat, high fiber, or high protein diets might work well for a short period of time, but because they typically deny you entire food groups, they are practically impossible to maintain for the long run.

In this question we will discuss the steps you need to take in order to eat healthily. Then, in Question 34 we will teach you what to do if you also need to lose weight. Since improved eating is such an important part of the *Heart♥SMART* program and a necessary part of your new, healthier life, we spoke to Teri Reilly, a registered dietitian, certified dietitian-nutritionist, certified diabetes educator. She is highly experienced and specializes in practical ways to helping people with heart disease and diabetes to lead a healthier, longer life.

Teri told us that there are three basic steps that will get you on the road to improving your health:

1. Get a game plan
2. Choose food wisely
3. Practice the *plate method* of portion control

As we discuss each step in detail, keep in mind that you will have a much better chance of being successful if you make small changes, a little at a time, rather than trying to make all the changes at once. Don't become discouraged if you struggle with some of the steps. Instead, focus on the changes that you are able to make and then feel proud of yourself for each little victory!

STEP 1: Get a Game Plan

Teri has many years of experience in helping people with heart disease to successfully make healthy changes to their lifestyle. She explains that planning is one of the most important parts of being successful. Some ways to plan successfully include

- Think about and plan your entire day of meals and snacks before the day begins. While this may not feel like fun or seem spontaneous, your heart and the rest of your body will thank you for trading spontaneity for health.
- Plan for and eat three meals and three snacks every day. When you eat frequently you will be less likely to be hungry, and your blood sugar level will remain steady throughout the day (which is important regardless of whether you are diabetic). When you aren't really hungry, you will be more likely to make healthier choices and less likely to eat junk food.
- Check out restaurant menus before you go there to make sure they have a healthy meal for you. Many restaurants post their menus online, and most are willing to modify menu options for special needs.
- Take meals and snacks with you to work or anywhere else that may not have healthy choices for you. Each time you plan a healthy meal or snack in advance, you give your body a chance to begin healing.

STEP 2: Choose Food Wisely

Teri explained there are foods that you should eat as a regular part of your life and foods that you should limit or avoid.

Eat These Foods

- **Whole grains** (foods that have the words whole wheat, bran, or grain as the first ingredient on the label): Unrefined, whole-grain foods contain fiber that can lower your blood cholesterol and your blood sugar. They can also help you to feel satisfied even when you eat smaller portions.
- **Healthy fats:** Despite what you may have learned, not all fats are bad for you. In fact, your body needs some fat to function

properly and to help you feel satisfied. The key is to eat all fats, including healthy ones, in moderation (pay attention to portion sizes), because although healthy, they are still very high in calories. Monounsaturated fat is a type of healthy fat. Canola oil and olive oil are two sources of monounsaturated fat, both of which can be used in cooking and salad dressings instead of other types of fats. Another source of monounsaturated fat is margarine that is free of trans-fats (and may lower your cholesterol), such as Benecol, Promise activ, or Smart Balance. Polyunsaturated fats are also heart healthy. These are found in nuts and seeds. When eaten in moderation, these may help lower your total blood cholesterol. Oily fishes also contain healthy fats called omega-3 fatty acids, and it is a good idea to eat these at least twice a week. Recent research shows that eating salmon, trout, and herring may help lower your risk of death from CAD.

- **Vegetables:** Teri recommends a variety of fresh vegetables and frozen vegetables should be a *large* part of your daily eating plan. Vegetables are rich in vitamins, full of fiber to keep you feeling satisfied, and contain phytochemicals (compounds that are found in vegetables, fruits, and whole grains that protect your cells from damage and reduce inflammation).Vegetables should be eaten raw or lightly cooked to preserve all their nutrients. They make great snacks and are easier to take along with you.

- **Fruit:** Like vegetables, fruit is low fat or fat free. They are rich in healthy nutrients and should be a significant part of your healthy eating program. Teri notes that if you have diabetes, you will need to limit your intake of fruit because it contains natural sugars.

- **Reduced-fat and fat-free dairy:** Dairy products (milk, cheeses, and yogurt) that are either fat free or contain less than 1 percent fat are an excellent source of protein in your heart healthy eating plan.

- **Lean meat, poultry, and vegetarian proteins:** Lean cuts of meat include chuck, sirloin, and tenderloin. White meat poultry (chicken and turkey) is the leanest and best choice. Ground meat or poultry should be the leanest possible (90 percent lean or higher). Be sure to remove any skin and fat before eating meat or poultry. Also, if necessary, prepare meat and poultry with healthy fats and avoid unhealthy saturated fats as additions to your meal. If you'd prefer to eat a vegetarian option, Teri recommends that one half cup of cooked legumes (black beans, kidney beans, white beans, pinto beans, black-eyed peas, and chickpeas) is a healthy portion of protein.

- **Fiber:** Foods that are rich in fiber should definitely be part of your new eating plan. Teri explained that the bottom line on fiber is that women need 25 grams a day and men need 38 grams a day. As we mentioned above, high fiber foods can lower your blood sugar levels and cholesterol. Dietary fiber also supports colon health. Good sources of fiber include oat bran, oatmeal, whole-grain breads and cereals, dried beans and peas (such as kidney beans, pinto beans, and black-eyed peas), fruits, and vegetables. If you have not been eating enough fiber, it is a good idea to increase the amount in your diet gradually in order to avoid digestive problems such as gas and bloating.

Limit or Avoid These Foods

- **Salt:** As we discussed in Question 30, salt will elevate your blood pressure, which can contribute to heart disease and increase your risk for heart attack. It is therefore important to limit the amount of salt you consume. Your goal is to eat less than 2,000 milligrams a day of salt (known as sodium). Begin by choosing not to add table salt to the foods you eat or prepare. Ask to have restaurant food prepared without salt. Reduce the amount of processed foods you consume, because these are typically very high in sodium. (Processed foods include many of those in boxes, cans, and bottles.) The nutrition facts label on all commercially prepared foods will indicate how many milligrams of salt are contained in the product.

- **Saturated fat:** Saturated fat raises your blood cholesterol levels, so limit or avoid foods that contain saturated fats. These foods include dairy products that have more than 1 percent fat, butter, shortening, lard, and tropical oils like palm and coconut. Also limit all cuts of meat and dairy that are not on the above list of lean meats and poultry. Unhealthy fats are also found in bacon fat, gravies, cream sauces, nondairy creamers, hydrogenated margarines, cocoa butter (found in chocolate), and cottonseed oil.

- **Partially hydrogenated oil:** This oil is considered extremely unhealthy because it contains trans fats, which raise your LDL cholesterol and lower your HDL cholesterol. Trans fats have been shown to significantly increase the risk for CAD. So read the labels on the foods you buy! If you see the words "partially hydrogenated oil," choose something else to eat. Many commercially prepared, packaged, and processed foods contain partially hydrogenated oil. You will find it in margarine, salad dressings, crackers, breads, cakes, cookies, granola bars, microwave popcorn, and prepared meals. This is another reason to limit the amount of processed foods that you eat. Soybean oil is the most commonly used partially hydrogenated oil. It's not nearly as healthy as its name might sound. Almost all fried foods contain partially hydrogenated oil (unless you know that they have been prepared with only canola or olive oil). In addition to looking for the words partially hydrogenated in the list of ingredients, you should also look at the nutrition facts label of all commercial prepared products for the presence of trans fats. Trans fats are considered such a serious health concern that they are now banned from many restaurants!

- **Cholesterol:** You should aim to eat less than 300 milligrams of cholesterol daily. The nutrition facts label on commercially prepared foods will tell you how much cholesterol is in that food. In general, foods low in saturated fats tend to be lower in cholesterol. In addition to the foods discussed in the saturated fat section, egg yolks also contain cholesterol and should be limited.

- **Sugar:** Too much sugar can cause weight gain and also increase your blood sugar levels. Most foods that are high in sugar are not rich in healthy nutrients and often contain trans fats (for example, cookies, cakes, muffins, granola bars, and chocolate). Others are fat free, but that doesn't make them healthy. Sugar-sweetened soda, hard and gummy candies, and sugary gum fall into this category. To complicate matters, it is also a good idea to limit diet drinks. They do not contain calories or sugar (so they seem ideal), but when you eat or drink sweet-tasting sugar-free foods and drinks, your body is tricked into believing you just consumed sugar. In response, your body will produce excess insulin. As you know, insulin is responsible for taking the sugar that circulates in your bloodstream and moving it into your cells. All that insulin will cause your blood sugar level to fall below a threshold, and you will become hungry and will eat more than your body really needs. This is the reason people don't lose weight despite switching to diet soda.

Note: Until you figure out exactly how to eat, all these dos and don'ts can seem overwhelming and confusing. To help you sort through it all, it can be very helpful to speak to a dietician who understands how to manage heart disease and can also help you develop an eating plan personalized to meet your calorie and nutrition requirements.

You might be interested to know that the U.S. health care system is beginning to recognize preventative medicine as an important tool in managing chronic diseases like hypertension (high blood pressure), heart disease, and diabetes. You should, therefore, check with your insurance plan, because you may have insurance coverage for medical nutrition therapy.

STEP 3: Practice the Plate Method of Portion Control

Teri told us that the plate method—recommended by many dieticians—is the best tool to ensure you are eating as healthily as possible at every meal. You should use the plate method whether you eat at home or at a restaurant. It is works like this:

- 50 percent of your plate should be filled with non-starchy vegetables (salad greens, carrots, cucumbers, peppers, beans, broccoli, cauliflower, brussels sprouts, and spinach). These are filling, low-calorie, and rich in phytochemicals, which reduce the inflammation that is associated with heart disease.
- 25 percent of your plate should be a healthy protein (low fat dairy, lean meat, fish, or legumes). Many people believe that when it comes to protein, more is better. But Teri told us that a serving of protein is about three ounces, which is about the size of your palm. You might want to purchase an inexpensive food scale to weigh foods until you can estimate portions well.
- 25 percent of your plate should be filled with a serving of whole grains (whole grain pasta, quinoa, or brown rice) or a starchy vegetable (a sweet or white potato). For the most part, a serving of starch is about half a cup. However, Teri explains that individual needs for starches can vary, depending on your energy and health needs. For example, for those who have diabetes, not having enough starches can also not be healthy. If you have diabetes or other health concerns that might be impacted by how you eat, it is always best to consult a dietician about your specific nutritional needs.

THE NITTY GRITTY

I know that eating fish is healthy,
but aren't there risks associated with eating too much fish?

As we have discussed, oily fish is rich in omega-3 fatty acids, spe-cifically the very long chain omega-3 polyunsaturated fatty acids, eicosapentaenoic acid (EPA), and docosahexaenoic acid (DHA). Eating two servings (about 6 to 8 ounces) a week of fish high in EPA and DHA is linked with a reduced risk of both sudden death and death from coronary heart disease in adults.[30] However, in recent years, findings have emerged demonstrating that certain fish are contaminated with high levels of mercury and other organic com-pounds. These are typically large fish that survive by eating other fish, causing them to ingest and accumulate larger amounts of mer-cury than fish that eat mainly plants. You can check with your local and state authorities to discover which types of fish may be contami-nated in your area. The Food and Drug Administration (FDA) also maintains a website with the most up-to-date recommendations for specific subpopulations in the United States (for example, chil-dren and pregnant women). For most people, however, when eaten within the guidelines established by the FDA and the Environmental Protection Agency (EPA), the benefits of eating fish far outweigh the potential risks—this includes adult men and postmenopausal women. In addition to regularly eating fish, there is some data that demonstrate that people with CAD may benefit from taking fish oil supplements. This may be especially helpful for people who have ele-vated triglyceride levels (another form of fat in the blood). Ask your doctor if you are a candidate for fish oil therapy. When you do use a supplement, a typical dose is 2 to 4 grams of EPA plus DHA per day.

I've heard something about the glycemic index. What is this and how can it help me?

The glycemic index (GI) ranks carbohydrates on a scale of 1 to 100 based on how quickly they raise blood sugar levels. The lower the number, the more slowly they raise blood sugar, and are therefore healthier. As you might imagine, foods high in sugar and refined flours have higher GI ratings. In Appendix A you can find GI resources.

The GI can help you make healthy food choices, but it is not a mandatory part of eating healthily. Some people find it confusing. If you find it confusing, simply stick to whole grain, low-sugar, low-fat foods, and manage your portions. You'll be fine!

Should I take supplements or vitamins?

The American Heart Association (AHA) recommends eating fruit and vegetables that are rich in antioxidants. However, while there is a great deal of evidence that diets rich in antioxidants (like the Mediterranean diet[31]) contribute to heart health, clinical studies[32] have not found antioxidant and vitamin supplementation in pill form to be beneficial. There is also no evidence to support the use of soy protein or isoflavone supplements instead of dairy or other proteins. Similarly, there does not seem to be a cardiovascular benefit from taking folate (folic acid) or other vitamin B supplements, despite its somewhat weak effect in lowering homocysteine levels, which have been associated with elevated CAD risk.

I heard that the DASH diet may help my heart. What is this diet?

The DASH diet is designed for people with high blood pressure, but it is a very good cardiac diet as well.[33] DASH stands for Dietary Approaches to Stop Hypertension, and studies have shown that patients on the DASH diet reduced their blood pressure within two weeks. The DASH diet requires a specific number of servings daily from various food groups. The number of servings you require will vary, depending on your caloric needs. You can learn more about the DASH diet by referring to the resources in Appendix 2.

QUESTION 34

Since having the angioplasty, Michael has been seriously contemplating his future, more specifically, his weight. He remembers he first discovered his heart disease when he began exercising—another of many attempts to lose weight. Now, Michael sees that he must make losing weight a priority. He wants to be alive to enjoy as much time as possible with his family, and he knows that losing weight is one of the most important parts of this battle. Michael wants to take every step to lose weight, but he's worried that he won't be successful because . . .

I've been battling my weight for years, and now my life depends on it. How am I supposed to lose weight now?

THE BOTTOM LINE

It can be very difficult to confront the fact that your weight is putting you at risk for heart disease, a heart attack, and possibly even death. For many people it is very hard to face the fact that they are overweight. In fact, it is quite common to tell yourself that your weight is fine even when you are not at a healthy weight. In most cases it is not a great idea to rely on your own perspective about your weight. Rather, you need an objective method for determining whether or not you need to lose weight. Then, if necessary, you need a plan for how to lose weight.

How do I know if my weight is healthy?

A healthy body weight is defined as a body mass index (BMI) of 18.5 to 24.9 (which is a measurement of kilograms per meter of height squared). You are overweight if your BMI is between 25 and 29.9 and obese if your BMI is 30 or more.

This number is extremely important, because a BMI of 30 or more has been shown to be a risk factor for CAD, even if you have no other risk factors. Excess body weight is a serious health risk, and it increases your risk for cardiovascular disease and for heart attack by increasing LDL cholesterol levels (bad cholesterol), triglyceride levels, blood pressure, and blood sugar levels. Extra body weight also reduces HDL cholesterol (good cholesterol). Therefore, *reaching and maintaining a healthy weight are critical components in reducing your risk for CAD.* There are a couple of ways to calculate your BMI. The first is to have a professional (a doctor, dietician, or an exercise specialist) calculate it for you. An even easier way is to use an online BMI calculator. You will find one listed in Appendix 2, so you can take this step right now!

I admit it. I'm overweight. What should I do right now?

To start, you should feel proud of yourself for admitting that you need to lose weight. This is the first step in making the important changes that will dramatically improve your quality of life and even lengthen it. We will offer several steps to help you achieve success, but these are the *five* that you should take right now. You might even find you will lose weight with these changes alone.

1. **Stop drinking extra calories** (sugar-sweetened soda, juice, wine, beer, liquor, energy drinks, and all other sugar-sweetened drinks). Research shows that drinking empty calories is one of

the top causes of weight gain in the United States. However, do not replace sugary drinks with diet drinks, because research shows that diet drinks don't necessarily help weight loss and may actually cause weight gain. Instead, replace sweetened drinks with water and seltzer. You might want to flavor your plain water with a squeeze of lemon, lime, or orange. Unsweetened iced tea is also a good choice.

2. **Don't skip meals!** Aim for at least three balanced meals (see Question 33) and one healthy snack. Many people try to jump-start their weight loss by skipping meals or snacks. In reality, this has the opposite effect, because when you do eventually eat, you will be really hungry and more likely to consume too many calories. Skipping meals also causes your blood sugar level to drop dramatically, which will make you more likely to choose less healthy carbohydrates that you can grab quickly.

3. **Set a weight loss goal.** We suggest that your first weight-loss goal be 10 percent of your current weight. Research shows that a 10 percent weight loss can have a noticeably positive impact on cholesterol levels, blood pressure, blood sugar levels, and general well-being. It may even reduce your doses of medications. After you have lost the first 10 percent, you can set another manageable goal. Simply setting the goal will help motivate you to make healthy changes.

4. **Increase your fiber intake.** Fiber keeps you feeling satisfied and helps you maintain a steady blood sugar level. The recommended daily intake for men is 30–35 grams and for women 25 grams.

5. **Begin an exercise program.** Make sure that you have medical clearance to exercise, and then start very slowly, especially if you have never exercised before. We suggest that you take a look at Question 32 in order to get going.

I think I can do it! What are my next steps?

As you probably know, it can be difficult to make the commitment to losing weight. Hopefully, now that your life may depend on it, you will feel a new level of dedication to your health. We offer you suggestions as to the steps you should take, but you will need to take these steps and stick with them for the rest of your life. We believe in you and want you to succeed, but if you feel you can't do it on your own, don't hesitate to seek help from a professional who understands what you need to succeed. The three types of professional support you might need are

1. A **registered dietician** to help you create and stick to a healthy eating plan that will result in weight loss.
2. An **exercise specialist** who will develop an exercise plan for your specific needs and fitness level. A fitness trainer can also work with you regularly to make sure that you are sticking with your program.
3. A **psychologist or counselor** can help you understand the emotional triggers that cause you to overeat or lose your motivation.

Now, you are really ready to lose weight. Here's what you need to know in order to continue making healthy changes that will result in weight loss. Let's do it!

1. You will have to figure out how many calories you need each day in order to maintain your current weight. Your doctor or dietician can help you with this information or you can find an online calculator online by using the search phrase "how many calories do I need." We have provided a resource for you in Appendix 2.
2. Once you have calculated your current calorie needs, you will be able to figure out what changes you need to make in order to lose weight.

3. Your goal is to create a deficit. You will only lose weight if you consume fewer calories than your body requires as energy.

4. One pound is equal to 3,500 calories. In order to lose one pound of body weight, you need to figure out how many calories create a deficit of 3,500 calories either by consuming less (reduce calorie intake) or by exercising more (burn off calories). Once you create the 3,500-calorie deficit, you will lose one pound.

5. Teri Reilly, our expert registered dietician, recommends that you should lose weight slowly in order to lose weight successfully and keep it off. Quick weight loss means that you made drastic changes to your lifestyle. This isn't healthy, and it is almost always too difficult to maintain in the long run. Weight loss is a marathon, not a sprint. To reach a healthy weight, make small changes a little at a time.

6. Teri suggests that you aim to create a deficit of 500 calories a day. That means 500 fewer calories than you need to maintain your current weight (not necessarily 500 fewer than you are currently consuming). Over the course of one week you will reduce your total calorie intake by 3,500 (7 x 500) and lose one pound. You can create the 500 calorie/day deficit by
   - **Eating/drinking 500 fewer calories.** You might be able to do this, but you may feel hungry.
   - **Burning off 500 calories through exercise.** This is very difficult to do and probably unrealistic for many people. (For example, you need to jog or run at 5 mph for one hour in order to burn about 500 calories.)
   - **A combination of eating less and exercising.** *This is our recommendation, and most likely to result in your success.* You can aim to burn off about 100 calories/one mile that you walk, and then consume less to make up the remaining calories.

7. Start reading nutrition labels carefully in order to determine the calories in the foods and drinks you consume. You will need to begin calculating how many calories you consume each day. You can do this by keeping track in a journal or by using an online

calorie-tracking program. You will find terrific web-based tools simply by searching for "free calorie tracking programs." These will track your calorie consumption, and many will include an exercise component. If you make some changes and don't lose weight, you need to reduce your calorie intake a bit more or increase your exercise (as long as you have the approval of your physician to do so).

8. In addition to aiming for a calorie deficit, be sure that you use all the suggestions in Question 33 for healthy eating. These give you the information you need to maintain a healthy lifestyle for the rest of your life.

THE NITTY GRITTY

Losing weight is not easy for most people, so don't be discouraged if you aren't able to reach your goals immediately. We can't stress enough that you should make slow changes, because the faster you lose the weight, the faster you will gain it back once you stop "dieting." Set small, realistic weight-loss goals. Share your goals with someone, because making your goals public can help you stick to them.

If you do find yourself eating in a way that you shouldn't, or if you skip a day (or a week) of exercise, don't give up. Instead, forgive yourself and simply start over. As long as you keep trying, then little by little you will reach your realistic eating and exercise goals. Once you reach your weight-loss goal, maintain it by following the suggestions in Question 33.

Here are a few quick tips to keep in mind as you work on your weight loss goal:

- **Eat more vegetables and fruits.** (If you are diabetic, ask your doctor how much fruit is recommended.)

- **Eat the right balance of protein.** Protein has the same amount of calories per gram as carbohydrates, so it is important to get some protein into your system, but not too much. Also, did you know that animal products are the primary source of saturated fats (the bad kind)? Teri tells us that this is because Americans usually choose red meat. Be sure to choose the healthiest sources of protein.
- **Eat enough healthy fats.** Cutting out fat completely is a weight-loss trend, but it isn't good for your body, and it will result in your feeling hungry, which means that you will overeat.

QUESTION **35** ——————————

Michael has made several changes to his lifestyle in order to become healthier and lose weight. He is walking on a treadmill three times a week (his goal is to add two more days over the next two months). He used to drink at least two glasses of sugar-sweetened soda a day, and now he has completely stopped drinking soda. Michael credits this as the reason he has already lost three pounds. In addition, he has switched to low-fat dairy and has significantly cut down on red meat, cookies, and—his favorite—cake. Michael continues to assess his diet because he knows he still has a long way to go. He is now considering alcohol. He enjoys a beer or a glass of wine a few times a week, so he is wondering . . .

Do I have to stop drinking alcohol when I start the Heart♥SMART program?

THE BOTTOM LINE

You may be surprised to learn that there isn't a clear-cut answer to this question. Rather, when you have coronary disease, the pros and cons of drinking alcohol depend on a couple of factors, and you must weigh these carefully in order to determine the best possible outcome for your health. To start, let's take a careful look at the two cons to drinking alcohol when you have heart disease.

Your experience with alcohol

This is the most important factor in determining your future relationship with alcohol. Research shows that small to moderate alcohol consumption is beneficial to your heart (more on this later). However, if you are a recovering alcoholic or if you have ever had a problem with alcohol that has caused you to stop drinking completely, *do not* start drinking again, no matter what research may suggest. The risks associated with drinking too much alcohol far outweigh any benefits to your heart. In addition, if, based on experience, you worry that you could become dependent on alcohol, don't start drinking now.

Your comfort level with drinking alcohol

Some people do not enjoy the taste of alcohol, no matter how it is mixed or disguised. If you are one of these, do not force yourself to drink simply because you have heard that it is "good" for your heart or because all your friends are doing it.

Some people don't like the altered-state feeling that alcohol creates. If you are very sensitive to the effect of alcohol or if it makes you feel too drunk or too relaxed, then don't feel compelled to drink any, regardless of what you may read or hear.

If you don't fall into either of these categories, you might be surprised to learn that consuming a modest amount of alcohol may actually be good for your heart. Research has found that for people who already have CAD, drinking a moderate amount of alcohol can significantly reduce their mortality (death) rate by 15 to 25 percent relative to nondrinkers who have CAD. In addition, you will be happy to know that drinking small amounts of alcohol is generally not a problem when mixed with most cardiac medications. However, there are a few exceptions, so if you take medications for heart disease or anything else, check with your doctor before consuming alcohol.

Can I drink as much as I want?

Several studies have evaluated the impact of alcohol consumption on heart health, and the findings are interesting and important. One study revealed that heavy drinkers have the highest rate of mortality (death), those who abstain (don't drink at all) have the second highest rate of mortality, while moderate drinkers have the lowest rate.[34] Another study found that light drinkers have about a 30 percent lower risk of developing CAD compared to lifelong abstainers, which then results in an approximately 10 percent lower overall risk of mortality.[35]

Moderate alcohol intake has also been associated with a decrease in sudden cardiac death in healthy adults. In a study of 85,067 women without reported cardiovascular disease, light-to-moderate alcohol consumption was associated with a 36 percent lower risk of sudden cardiac death when compared to those who abstained from alcohol. Another study of 22,071 male physicians showed that men who consumed light-to-moderate amounts of alcohol (two to six drinks per week) had up to an 80 percent lower risk of sudden cardiac death when compared to nondrinkers. This compelling research confirms that modest alcohol consumption can have some health benefits.

How does drinking a small amount of alcohol reduce the risk of cardiovascular disease?

Scientists have not yet fully uncovered the reasons why alcohol supports heart health, but there are some plausible biological explanations for it. The most compelling of these possible reasons is that alcohol can substantially increase HDL (good) cholesterol levels. Some researchers believe that an increase in HDL may be responsible for up to 50 percent of alcohol's beneficial effects on CAD. In fact, research has shown that moderate drinking increased HDL by about 12 percent, which is similar to the increase seen with some medications and with exercise programs. Furthermore, moderate alcohol consumption has also been associated with a reduction in LDL (bad) cholesterol. Finally, it has been shown that drinking alcohol can reduce the tendency of blood clot formation that can lead to heart attacks. In the medical literature, this is called an *antithrombotic effect*.[36]

What exactly does "moderate" mean?

Research finds that there appears to be an optimal dose of alcohol consumption that might improve heart health or assist in slowing progression of the disease. This amount is reflected in a J-curve relationship between alcohol consumption and mortality. More specifically, the ideal amount of alcohol consumption appears to be between one-half to one drink per day.

How much is "a drink"?

One drink refers to a 12-ounce bottle of beer, a 5-ounce glass of wine, or 1.5 ounces of liquor (either alone or in a mixed drink). That being said, it is important to include any alcohol (and mixers) as part of your daily caloric intake. If you work with a dietician, be sure to share your alcohol consumption.

Remember that this recommendation is for *one* drink *per* day. Drinking several servings of alcohol in one day is *not* the same as drinking one a day. In fact, drinking this much at one time can be dangerous for your health.

What could happen if I drink too much?

Drinking too much alcohol is associated with several possible diseases specifically related to consuming too much alcohol. These include

- Liver damage
- Internal bleeding
- Alcoholic cardiomyopathy (weakening of the heart muscle, possibly leading to congestive heart failure)
- High blood pressure
- Increased rates of hemorrhagic stroke (bleeding in the brain that leads to a stroke)
- Some types of arrhythmias (abnormal heart rhythms)

Research supports these concerns. In fact, one study found that when people drank more than six alcoholic beverages a day, their risk for sudden death more than doubled.

THE NITTY GRITTY

I've heard people talk about the French paradox. What is this?

The French paradox refers to the fact that France has a low rate of coronary disease despite a high prevalence of the usual risk factors and a diet rich in saturated fats. Research has revealed that, in fact, mortality (death) is actually lower for those countries that have a culture of drinking wine (like France) compared to countries where beer or liquor are the predominant alcoholic beverages. Following this distinction, a great deal of research sought to determine whether the cardiovascular benefits of drinking alcohol are actually confined to wine, specifically red wine. So far, several nonalcoholic compounds in red wine have been identified and determined to be beneficial. In particular, phenolic compounds are credited with having antioxidant and antithrombotic properties. The most well known of the phenolic compounds is resveratrol, which has been associated with lower incidences of cancer and cardiovascular disease as well as cholesterol-lowering and anti-inflammatory properties. In the 1990s, this research caused red wine sales in the United States to skyrocket, and these sales continue to remain high.

Research with respect to resveratrol is ongoing; however, newer studies suggest that the majority of the benefit is due to the alcohol rather than the compounds specific to red wine. Therefore, modest consumption of any type of alcohol on a regular basis is likely to be associated with similar benefits.

I've heard that drinking alcohol can cause breast cancer. Is that true?

There is research that supports a relationship between alcohol consumption and breast cancer. From 1980 to 2008, researchers conducted a study of the health of 105,986 nurses—the famous Nurses' Health Study. A part of this research studied the women's alcohol consumption.[37] They found that women who consumed three to six drinks of alcohol per week had a 15 percent increased risk of breast cancer. Even more striking was the finding that women who consumed two drinks per day had a more than 50 percent greater risk of breast cancer when compared with women who did not drink at all. The type of alcohol consumed did not make a difference.

Since these findings are not insignificant, each woman must weigh this slightly higher risk of breast cancer against the positive effects on heart disease of drinking small quantities of alcohol. One factor to consider is your personal and family history of each disease. Another factor is the general risk of getting either of these diseases. Most notably, only one in twenty-five women die of breast cancer, while at least one in three die of cardiovascular disease, such as heart attack and stroke. Therefore, the benefits of drinking a small amount of alcohol may well outweigh the risk of breast cancer for most women. Before making a final decision, it is important to discuss your personal benefits and risks with your doctor.

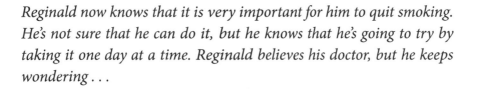

Q U E S T I O N **36**

Reginald now knows that it is very important for him to quit smoking. He's not sure that he can do it, but he knows that he's going to try by taking it one day at a time. Reginald believes his doctor, but he keeps wondering . . .

I know smoking can cause cancer, but what does it have to do with my heart?

THE BOTTOM LINE

Almost everyone knows that smoking can cause lung cancer, and you may even know that it also *increases* your risk for every other type of cancer. However, cancer is not the only way that smoking can hurt you. There are toxic chemicals in cigarette smoke that can harm nearly every part of your body. In the United States, smoking is responsible for nearly one in five deaths. For example, smoking can cause *abdominal aortic aneurysms,* which is a weakening of the body's main artery (the aorta). This can lead to a rupture of the aorta and sudden death. Smoking is also a major risk factor for *peripheral vascular disease* (PVD), which can lead to blockages in the blood vessels outside the heart (such as the carotid artery and vessels in the legs). In addition, men who smoke are more likely to develop erectile dysfunction (impotence) resulting from blockages and dysfunction of their blood vessels. Statistics show that about half of all smokers who keep smoking will die from an illness related to smoking.

How does smoking affect my heart?

About 8.6 million people suffer from smoking-related lung *and* heart diseases. While most people associate cigarette smoking with breathing problems and lung cancer, you might be surprised to learn that in the United States that 20 to 30 percent of all deaths from heart disease are directly related to cigarette smoking. More specifically, smokers are two to four times more likely to get CAD than non-smokers, and their risk of dying from heart disease is two to three times higher. In addition, smokers are *twice* as likely to die from a heart attack than nonsmokers. By now, you clearly see that smoking is a major risk factor for developing CAD.

I believe the statistics, but how exactly does smoking cause heart disease?

There are substances in tobacco smoke, such as nicotine and carbon monoxide, which are highly toxic to blood vessels and can trigger CAD development. There are several ways in which these toxins impact your heart:

- *Smoking damages blood vessels.* As we mentioned in Question 5, smoking can damage the inner layer of blood vessels known as the endothelium. The endothelium functions to promote the health of blood vessels in several ways, the most important of which is to produce nitric oxide. Nitric oxide regulates blood flow by causing the blood vessels to properly dilate (open up and allow greater blood flow). Smoking can cause severe damage to the endothelial layer, which results in decreased nitric oxide production. When this happens, blood vessels can lose many important functions. They can become more vulnerable to developing cholesterol deposits, and blood clots are more readily able to form in the vessels (which may cause a heart attack).

- *Smoking changes blood platelets.* Smoking causes the platelets in your blood to clump together more easily, which will make the platelets more sticky and more likely to form blood clots. This will also increase the risk of a heart attack.

- *Smoking narrows arteries.* Smoking can cause your coronary arteries to spasm (narrow), which reduces the blood flow to the heart muscle.

- *Smoking causes cardiac arrhythmias.* Smoking can trigger the development of many types of irregular heartbeats, called arrhythmias. These can be dangerous for your heart.

- *Smoking causes atherosclerosis.* Smoking lowers HDL (good) cholesterol, which permits cholesterol-carrying lipoproteins in the blood to more easily penetrate the walls of the arteries, where they can then develop into a hard plaque and atherosclerosis.

- *Smoking reduces the amount of oxygen in your body.* The high concentration of carbon monoxide in tobacco smoke makes it difficult for red blood cells to carry the oxygen they need. Therefore, the amount of oxygen in your bloodstream is reduced.

Why is nicotine so harmful?

As mentioned above, cigarette smoke negatively affects your health in many ways. It is bad for your heart, blood vessels, hormones, metabolism, and brain. However, in addition to being extremely unhealthy, the nicotine in tobacco is as addictive as heroin or cocaine. Since nicotine occurs naturally in tobacco, a smoker quickly becomes addicted to the nicotine and to smoking. In fact, over time,

smokers become both physically addicted to nicotine and emotionally dependent upon it. The nicotine in tobacco is so powerful that
regular smoking for only a few weeks can lead to withdrawal symptoms when smoking is stopped suddenly. Since tobacco addiction
has both a physical and an emotional component, each attempt to
stop causes acute physical withdrawal symptoms as well as a strong
psychological need for the tobacco.

If you have ever tried to quit smoking you probably know the
symptoms of withdrawal start within a few hours of the last cigarette
and peak two to three days after quitting, because this is when most
of the nicotine and its by-products have been eliminated from your
body. Withdrawal symptoms can last from a few days to up to several weeks. They can include any of the following symptoms, but not
necessarily all of them:

- Dizziness (which may only last a day or two after quitting)
- Irritability
- Frustration, impatience, or anger
- Anxiety
- Difficulty concentrating or restlessness
- Headaches
- Fatigue
- Increased appetite or weight gain
- Sleep problems (trouble falling or staying asleep, bad dreams or
  nightmares)
- Sadness or depression
- Cough, dry mouth, sore throat, or postnasal drip

You may feel and truly believe that smoking calms you when you
are anxious or nervous. In reality, smoking does *not* reduce anxiety or stress. The nervous or restless feelings you may experience,
paired with a craving for a cigarette to calm you down, are actually symptoms of nicotine withdrawal. Conversely to what you may
believe, research shows that quitting smoking actually contributes to

lowering stress levels.[38] For highly dependent smokers who reported that smoking helped them cope with stress, smoking cessation was associated with lowered stress. While you may perceive a lowered stress level when you smoke a cigarette, in the long run, smoking may generate or aggravate negative emotional states such as stress or anxiety. The results of this study should reassure you that quitting smoking will not actually deprive you of a coping resource.

So it's hard to quit, but is it really worth it?

As you likely know, there are many benefits associated with not smoking. One of these important benefits is that your risk for developing CAD will drop quickly after you stop smoking. According to the World Health Organization, after one year of not smoking, a former smoker's risk of coronary artery disease decreases by 50 percent. In addition, your risk of having a heart attack decreases when you stop smoking[39], although, it takes about fifteen years after quitting to return to the same risk level for developing CAD as that of a nonsmoker.

If you have CAD and have had an angioplasty procedure or bypass surgery, it is even more important for you to quit smoking. Studies show that if you continue to smoke after having angioplasty or bypass surgery, you may not receive the full benefit from either of these procedures. The data consistently shows that the risk of death is higher for smokers than for those who are able to quit.[40]

What's the best way to quit?

There are many different ways to try to stop smoking and many philosophies as to which is the best way to do so. Most smokers have tried to quit many times. In fact, it may take a number of attempts until one is successful.

One of the best ways to quit is to attend a program. Smoking cessation programs can provide the support and advice that many people need in order to stop smoking permanently. However, it is important to choose the right program, because not all programs are equally effective. Look for a program that includes multiple sessions, because single-session programs almost never work. You should expect a high-quality program to include sessions of at least thirty minutes several times a week for a minimum of two weeks. There is strong evidence that the more intense (longer and more frequent) the treatment, the greater your chance of succeeding. In addition, it is important to make sure that the leader of the program you attend is thoroughly trained in smoking cessation.

In addition to attending a program, you might also want to join Nicotine Anonymous (NicA), a twelve-step program like Alcoholics Anonymous, which is designed to help you quit and stick with it.

We suggest you use caution before signing up for a program that promises results with a single session, a special pill, secret injections, charges a very high fee, or guarantees a 100 percent success rate. You should also exercise caution when a program does not want to provide references of people who have attended the program.

Can I use nicotine replacement therapy to help me quit?

When you try to stop smoking, using nicotine patches or another form of medical nicotine may help alleviate some of your physical withdrawal from nicotine so that you are able to focus on the psychological (emotional) aspects of quitting. However, since nicotine replacement only addresses the physical aspect of the addiction, you will still need other ways to tackle the psychological (emotional) parts of smoking. By also attending a smoking cessation program, you will be sure to address the emotional aspects as well. If you choose to use any form of nicotine replacement, make sure you stop smoking first! It is not safe to continue smoking and use nicotine replacement. In fact, the FDA has not approved any of these products for use in conjunction with tobacco. You risk a nicotine overdose, which can have serious consequences for your heart and your blood circulation.

Is it safe to use nicotine replacement if I already have CAD?

In 2000, the US Agency for Healthcare Research and Quality (AHRQ) Clinical Practice Guideline on Smoking Cessation issued a warning against the use of nicotine replacement for individuals with heart or circulatory diseases. However, the most recent 2008 Clinical Practice Guidelines determined that, when a physician carefully monitors use, nicotine patches can safely be used even by people with CAD. Therefore, if you are thinking of using any form of nicotine replacement, be sure to receive medical clearance from your doctor. Many physicians believe that, for some people with CAD, the benefits of quitting smoking outweigh the potential health risks of nicotine replacement. If you and your doctor agree that it is safe for you to try a nicotine patch, make sure you don't smoke a single cigarette while using the patches!

Can prescription drugs help me quit?

Several prescription drugs are designed to help you quit smoking, but as with nicotine replacement, they are best used in conjunction with another method, such as a support program. The two most commonly prescribed medications include

- **Bupropion (Zyban),** an antidepressant that acts on chemicals in the brain related to nicotine craving. Since bupropion does not contain nicotine, some doctors may recommend a combination therapy for heavily addicted smokers, such as bupropion along with a nicotine patch. For some people, this combination is more effective than using a single treatment alone.
- **Varenicline (Chantix)** is the newest medication developed to help people stop smoking. It works by interfering with nicotine receptors in the brain. Varenicline decreases the pleasurable effects of smoking and reduces the symptoms of nicotine withdrawal. It is, therefore, possible to begin taking this medication

and continue smoking for a few days before quitting. This can alleviate the psychological fear and stress of quitting cold turkey. Several studies have shown that varenicline more than doubles the chances of quitting smoking when compared to taking no medication at all.

Can I use natural methods to quit?

There are several methods that you might consider as part of your overall plan to quit smoking. For the most part, these address your emotional dependence on smoking and have different levels of success.

- **Hypnosis.** Most studies that have assessed the effectiveness of hypnosis have not supported it as a successful method. However, there are people who might find it useful. There are several variations of hypnosis, so you may want to try more than one kind to determine whether it may be effective for you.
- **Acupuncture.** Acupuncture for smoking is typically administered on certain parts of the ears. That being said, there is little scientific evidence to demonstrate that acupuncture helps you stop smoking.
- **Cold laser therapy.** This treatment is similar to acupuncture except a laser is used. The treatment is supposed to relax the smoker and trigger the release of endorphins (pain-relief substances that are made naturally by the body) in order to mimic the effects of nicotine in the brain. Currently there is no scientific evidence to demonstrate that this therapy helps people stop smoking.
- **Herbal therapy and supplements.** There is no scientific evidence to support the use of homeopathic aids and herbal supplements as a method to stop smoking. These formulations are considered dietary supplements, not medications, and as such, they do not need FDA approval in order to be sold to the public. As a

consumer, you should know that this means the manufacturers of these products do not have to provide any evidence that they work or even that they are safe. We suggest that you carefully read the label of any product that claims it can help you stop smoking. That being said, since the supplement industry is not regulated, a label may not be accurate. We strongly caution you against using any supplement without your doctor's approval of every ingredient it contains.

- **Electronic cigarettes.** In 2004 a Chinese company started making an electronic cigarette that looks like a cigarette, right down to the glowing tip. The electronic cigarette is sold with flavorings and with cartridges that contain different doses of nicotine, from high doses to no nicotine at all. When the smoker puffs on the cigarette, the system delivers a mist of liquid, resembling smoke, composed of nicotine and flavoring. This smoke is inhaled, delivering nicotine to the lungs. This mechanism is designed to address the physical addiction by providing nicotine as well as emotional dependence by mimicking the feeling of actual smoking. Over time, the smoker should wean himself off nicotine by using lower-dose cartridges, until eventually smoking the cigarette without any nicotine at all. While some smokers have had success with this technique, to date there is no published research proving it is a successful way to stop smoking. In addition, there are questions as to the safety of inhaling some of the substances used in electronic cigarettes. In most instances, the manufacturers of electronic cigarettes do not list the ingredients. Of course, they attest to the ingredients being safe; however, it is not clear whether, in fact, they are safe to inhale. For example, some substances might be safe to eat but could still harm the delicate tissues inside the lungs. In 2009 the FDA tested eighteen samples of cartridges from two leading electronic cigarette brands. They found cancer-causing substances in half the samples.

THE NITTY GRITTY

What is the success rate of quitting for good?

On any one attempt, only about 4 to 7 percent of smokers are able to quit smoking without medication or some other help. Based on clinical studies, when an attempt to quit is combined with medication, this number increases to about 25 percent. In addition, when combined with medication, counseling or other types of emotional support can further boost success rates.

Will I gain weight when I stop smoking?

Unfortunately, many smokers gain weight when they quit smoking, although the average weight gain is typically less than ten pounds. Women tend to gain slightly more weight than men do, and it appears that smokers gain weight when they quit even if they do not eat more. Some people are reluctant to try quitting, because they are afraid that they will gain weight. They even point to the health hazards of being overweight as a reason not to quit. However, you should know that the risks associated with continued tobacco use are far worse than the risks associated with gaining a bit of weight. As you try to quit smoking, you should not allow yourself to focus on the potential weight gain. If necessary, you can address your weight issues at a later point. In addition, consider the idea that exercise may be a good distraction from smoking *and* also prevent you from gaining weight.

A Final Word

Michael, Reginald, Rosa, Brian, and Diane have all come a long way since first being diagnosed with heart disease. Each has faced the initial anxiety of having a variety of diagnostic procedures, and each has had to cope with learning the diagnosis: heart disease. Their treatments have been somewhat different because each person's diagnosis required a slightly different medical intervention. They have all learned the value of taking prescribed medications, and they have all leaned the steps that they *must* take in order to become healthier and to reduce the chance that their heart disease will get worse. Michael, Reginald, Rosa, Brian, and Diane have all committed to making important changes that can dramatically improve their health, including eating more healthily, exercising, quitting smoking, and reducing stress. They have all come a long way, and each one continues to work toward improving his or her health a little more each day. They are motivated by wanting to live for as long as possible to experience all the riches that life has to offer.

Now that you have finished reading about our five friends, we have one last question for you: **Are you ready to make a commitment to taking care your health?** Your answer must be "yes." You are worth it and you have a lot to live for. We ask you to think about what in your life is most important to you. Write down your inspiration and always carry it with you.

As you now know, heart disease is chronic, and there is a good chance that your heart will develop more blockages if you do not take the necessary steps to prevent the progression of the disease. Having an angioplasty procedure or bypass surgery and taking medication are tremendously important. They are the first steps toward repairing the damage to your heart. You can reduce the possibility of needing further intervention by closely following all your doctor's recommendations, taking your medications as prescribed, following up with all medical visits, and by following the *Heart*♥SMART program.

You can do it! Take small steps until you are addressing all the changes necessary to ensure you a life that is as long and healthy as possible.

We wish you a full life filled with health, family, and friends,

Dr. Allen Jeremias and *Dr. Susan Bartell*

CPR Instructions

What exactly is "CPR"?

CPR stands for cardiopulmonary resuscitation, and it is an emergency procedure that is performed on someone who experiences cardiac arrest, which means that the person's heart is not pumping properly, so blood is not circulating. A bystander administers CPR in an attempt to temporarily simulate the pumping heart in order to circulate enough blood to preserve the brain until the heart begins working again and circulation is restored.

When someone has been diagnosed with heart disease or has had a heart attack, it is a good idea for family and friends to learn the basics of CPR in case an emergency situation arises that would require it. This does not mean that the person will die without receiving it; however, it is one of the many precautions that one should consider taking to protect a loved one. *CPR is performed on someone who is unresponsive and without any obvious signs of breathing or a heartbeat (pulse).* Below is a five-step guide to administering CPR. These instructions **do not** apply to trauma victims (after a car accident or a drowning) or to children, for whom different conditions must be met.

1. **Check:** To begin, if the victim is in an unsafe environment or location, if possible move him to a safe location and place him on his back. Before attempting CPR, make sure the person is not responding and does not have a pulse. Typically, a nonresponsive person will not respond to verbal stimulation (calling his name) or to physical stimulation (shaking him). In addition, there will

be no signs of breathing or the breathing will be agonal (which means nonproductive or labored). The person will not have a pulse. The best place to check a pulse is on the neck, just under the angle of the jawbone, where you would find the carotid artery. Take a moment to find and check your own carotid pulse so you know where it is and what it should feel like.

2. **Call:** *Before* you begin administering CPR, call 911. It is absolutely critical to ensure that help is on the way before you do anything else. The more quickly fully trained paramedics get to the scene, the more likely the victim will survive a cardiac arrest. Through CPR administration you will do your best to get the victim's blood pumping, but the chest compressions that you administer are unlikely to restore heart function. In most cases of cardiac arrest, the heart is in a very fast rhythm (called ventricular fibrillation). This rhythm is much too fast for the heart to be properly contracting in order to eject blood out of the heart. The most effective way to convert the heart back into a regular rhythm is by providing an electrical shock with a device called a defibrillator. The emergency responders carry this machine with them. CPR is administered not to convert the heart back to a regular rhythm but to provide a certain amount of blood circulation to the body (mainly the brain) and to bridge the time until the heart is defibrillated. This is why it is so critical to call 911 immediately. In addition, when you call, the dispatcher can assist you in assessing the victim and may also be able to guide you through the steps of CPR.

3. **Pump:** As soon as you have called 911, return to the victim, and if she is still unresponsive, begin administering chest compressions. First, make sure she is lying on her back on a hard surface, with her arms down to the sides. Don't do chest compressions on a bed, because you won't be able to compress the chest against the low resistance of the soft mattress. Next, find the center of the chest just above the stomach area, on the lower part of the breastbone. Place both hands on the chest. Keep your arms

straight and locked, with your body directly above the victim. Now begin to pump on the chest hard and fast at a rate of about 100 pushes a minute (faster than one a second). These pushes are called compressions. When you begin compressions, move your whole body up and down. Make sure you compress the breast-bone in about two inches and then let it out before beginning the next compression. The American Heart Association refers to the beat of the Bee Gees' song "Stayin' Alive" as an ideal rhythm to maintain the speed required. Give thirty compressions at a time. Don't worry about causing injury or harm—good chest com-pressions may break some ribs! In addition, don't worry about checking the person's pulse. Simply concentrate on giving com-pressions and providing breaths. (See Step 4.)

4. **Check airway:** After the first thirty compressions, stop and open the person's mouth to make sure there is nothing in his mouth or throat that could cause him to choke. If there is, remove it. If you are confident that he was not eating or that there is no other reason he may have choked, you may skip this step.

5. **Blow:** Tilt her head back and lift her chin up. Pinch her nose closed and cover her mouth with your mouth. Blow air into her mouth until you see her chest rise. Give two breaths. Each breath should take one second, which means you should not blow too fast. The ratio of chest compressions to rescue breaths is thirty to two, which means that you should administer thirty chest compressions followed by two breaths. Once you have delivered the two breaths, return immediately to the chest com-pressions. Continue this cycle until help arrives.

If two people are administering CPR, the cycle is exactly the same. When two-person CPR is administered, one person pumps the chest thirty times then stops to allow the other person to administer the two mouth-to-mouth breaths. After the second person administers the two breaths, the first person gives thirty compressions again, and the CPR team continues in this way.

What complications can occur while I'm conducting CPR?

Vomiting is the most frequently encountered complication of CPR. If the victim starts to vomit, turn his head to the side and try to sweep out or wipe off the vomit. Continue administering CPR.

Can I get an infection when giving CPR?

The spread of infection from the victim to the rescuer is exceedingly rare. Most cardiac arrests occur in people's homes, so relatives or friends will likely administer CPR. In addition, even when CPR is performed on strangers, there is an extremely small risk of infection. There is **NO** documentation of HIV or AIDS ever having been transmitted via CPR.

Can I do chest compressions only?

Compression-only CPR is a technique that involves chest compressions without artificial respiration (mouth-to-mouth breathing). Most recent research shows that untrained rescuers tend to be more comfortable with this simple method because it is easier to administer. In addition, findings show that bystanders are more likely to help a victim when they do not have to administer mouth-to-mouth breathing. It is notable that the survival rate for chest compressions-only CPR is similar to the survival rate for traditional CPR.

Can CPR alone restart the heart?

As we mentioned above, CPR alone is unlikely to restart the heart. The main purpose of this rescue technique is to restore the partial flow of oxygenated blood to the brain and heart. The goal of CPR is to delay tissue death and to extend the brief window of opportunity for a successful resuscitation without permanent brain damage. Administration of an electric shock to the subject's heart (defibrillation) is usually needed in order to restore a viable or perfusing heart rhythm.

APPENDIX TWO

Resources

General Health

Centers for Disease Control and Prevention
http://www.cdc.gov
Information on a range of diseases as well as resources to quit smoking.

National Institute on Aging
http://www.nia.nih.gov
A national organization promoting health, fitness, and wellness for older adults.

ShareCare
http://www.sharecare.com
An interactive website that provides users with accurate information about health and connects them with experts and other users in order to educate, empower, and continue the conversations of health.

WebMD
http://www.webmd.com
A comprehensive health information website offering in-depth, accurate information on a wide range of topics as well as an online community to which all users can contribute.

World Health Organization
http://www.who.int/en
An international organization focused on global public health issues.

Heart Health

American Heart Association
http://www.heart.org
A national nonprofit organization whose mission is to raise awareness of heart disease. The website includes a "Getting Healthy" section with information on both nutrition and exercise.

Adult Congenital Heart Association
http://www.achaheart.org/
Extensive information designed to educate both ACHD patients and health care professionals about the special needs of adults with heart defects.

AF Stat: A Call to Action for Atrial Fibrillation
https://www.afstat.com
A collaboration of health care leaders and organizations working to improve the health and well-being of people affected by atrial fibrillation (AFib).

American Association of Cardiovascular and Pulmonary Rehabilitation
http://www.aacvpr.org
A multidisciplinary professional association comprised of health professionals who serve in the field of cardiac and pulmonary rehabilitation. AACVPR provides an online directory of cardiac rehabilitation programs that can be searched by state.

British Heart Foundation
http://www.bhf.org.uk
Britain's nonprofit organization whose mission is to raise awareness of heart health and prevention of heart disease.

CardioSmart
http://www.cardiosmart.org
The patient education and support program launched by the American College of Cardiology.

Clinical Trial Results
http://www.clinicaltrialresults.org
Comprehensive website featuring summaries of current and past cardiovascular disease clinical trials.

Heart Rhythm Society
http://www.hrsonline.org
An international nonprofit organization that promotes education and advocacy for cardiac arrhythmia professionals and patients. It provides readers with information about arrhythmias, devices, and cardiovascular electrophysiology.

Heart to Heart
http://brucejohnsonhearttoheart.com
Bruce Johnson, a veteran broadcast journalist in Washington, DC, wrote *Heart to Heart* after he survived a massive heart attack at age forty-two.

The Heart Truth
http://www.nhlbi.nih.gov/educational/hearttruth
A national heart disease awareness campaign for women, supported by the National Heart, Lung and Blood Institute.

Hearts in Harmony
http://www.healthyheartsinharmony.com
Information for heart survivors about the physical and often overlooked emotional aspects of recovering from a heart event.

Hypertrophic Cardiomyopathy Association
http://www.4hcm.org
A not-for-profit organization that provides information, support, and advocacy to patients, their families, and medical providers.

Mended Hearts, Inc
http://mendedhearts.org/
A national nonprofit organization that provides support and education to heart disease patients, families, and caregivers.

National Heart, Lung and Blood Institute
http://www.nhlbi.nih.gov
Heart disease information for patients and their families, including the DASH Diet.

PedHeart Resource
http://heartpassport.com
Clinical descriptions of heart defects, treatment information, tutorials, and PDF patient handouts. Slides and image libraries are also available.

Preventive Cardiovascular Nurses Association
http://www.pcna.net
A leading nursing organization dedicated to preventing cardiovascular disease through assessing risk, facilitating lifestyle changes, and guiding individuals to achieve treatment goals.

SecondsCount
http://www.secondscount.org
An extensive patient website created by the Society for Cardiovascular Angiography and Interventions. It offers information on cardiovascular disease, procedures, treatments, and tools for living a healthy life.

Speak from the Heart
http://www.speakfromtheheart.com
This site includes videos from real patients telling their angina stories, separating angina facts from myths, angina animation, and a personal assessment for patients to complete and share with their cardiologists.

StentPlus+
http://www.stentplus.com
Information for patients who have received a drug-eluting stent.

StopAfib.org
http://www.stopafib.org
A patient-to-patient resource to help you control atrial fibrillation so it doesn't control your life.

Sudden Cardiac Arrest Association (SCCA)
http://associationdatabase.com
Nonprofit organization focused on sudden cardiac arrest. SCAA identifies and unites survivors, those at risk of sudden cardiac arrest, and others who are interested in being advocates on SCAA issues in their communities and beyond.

Time to Talk Cardio
http://timetotalkcardio.com
Program to help patients and health care professionals make the most of their conversations by building communication skills to help better manage heart health.

Women's Health

Food and Drug Administration Office of Women's Health
http://www.fda.gov,
then search "heart health for women"
Consumer information regarding women's heart health.

PFO Research Foundation
http://pforesearch.org
Seeks to educate the public about patent foramen ovale (PFO) and support research into the condition's related disorder.

Sister to Sister: The Women's Heart Health Foundation
http://www.sistertosister.org
A foundation devoted to women's heart health, including acquiring information, finding support, and taking action.

U.S. Department of Health and Human Services Office on Women's Health
http://www.womenshealth.gov
A site devoted to women's health issues, including specific information about recognizing and surviving a heart attack.

WomenHeart: The National Coalition for Women with Heart Disease
http://www.womenheart.org
A patient advocacy group whose mission is to improve the quality of life and health of women living with or at risk of heart disease and to advocate for their benefit.

US Against Athero
http://www.usagainstathero.com
A national effort to spread awareness of atherosclerosis. Learn more about what steps you can take to slow the progression of atherosclerosis.

Minorities Health

Health Power for Minorities
A website dedicated to improving the health of multicultural, racial, and ethnic minority populations or minority populations.

Healthy Eating and Nutrition

BMI Calculator
www.nhlbisupport.com/bmi
This National Institute of Health (NIH) BMI calculator makes it easy for you to calculate your body fat using your height and weight (English or metric).

Dietary Guidelines for Americans
http://health.gov/dietaryguidelines
Advice for people two years and older about how good dietary habits can promote health and reduce risk for major chronic diseases.

Eatright.org
http://www.eatright.org
Website by the Academy of Nutrition and Dietetics. An excellent resource for evidence-based nutrition information.

Fruits and Vegetables More Matters
http://www.fruitsandveggiesmorematters.org
An explanation of the USDA's updated dietary guidelines.

Glycemic Index
http://www.glycemicindex.com
The *Glycemic Index* (GI) is a numerical scale used to indicate how fast and how high a particular food can raise your blood glucose (blood sugar) level. Lower GI foods are generally healthier.

Healthy Dining Finder
http://www.healthydiningfinder.com
A guide to American restaurants and a resource for the healthiest menu selections, including accurate nutritional information for menu selections.

Produce for Better Health Foundation
http://www.pbhfoundation.org
Information about fruits and vegetables and how to incorporate them into every occasion.

SparkPeople
http://www.sparkpeople.com
A diet and health website focused on helping you begin a healthy lifestyle and a weight loss plan.

U.S. Food and Drug Administration
http://www.fda.gov
Offers the definitions of nutrient claims allowable by the FDA and an explanation and guide to the food nutrition label required to be on all food items.

USDA Choose My Plate
http://www.choosemyplate.gov
Basic meal planning according to the food groups, this plan replaces the food pyramid.

USDA Nutrient Database
http://ndb.nal.usda.gov
A resource to identify the nutritional data of manufactured food.

Physical Activity

American College of Sports Medicine
http://www.acsm.org
International organization promoting the advancement of health through science, education, and medicine.

Couch to 5K Running Program
http://www.coolrunning.com
A beginner's guide to becoming healthy by initiating an individual running program.

Healthways Silver Sneakers Fitness Program for Older Adults
http://www.silversneakers.com
A health, exercise, and wellness program helping older adults live healthy, active lifestyles.

U.S. Department of Health and Human Services, 2008 Physical Activity Guidelines for Americans
http://www.health.gov/paguidelines
Science-based, physical activity guidelines for Americans aged six and older.

Diabetes

American Diabetes Association
http://www.diabetes.org
Information about diabetes, its symptoms, and preventive and postdiagnostic lifestyle tips.

Stress Reduction

American Institute of Stress
http://www.stress.org
A nonprofit organization and website to help you understand stress and its role in health and illness.

American Psychological Association
http://www.apa.org
A national organization covering a wide range of topics related to emotional and physical health, including stress reduction. It includes a search engine to find a licensed psychologist.

HelpGuide
http://helpguide.org
Expert, advertising-free information resources for all aspects of health challenges, including stress.

Quit Smoking

American Lung Association
http://www.lung.org
1-866-QUIT-YES (1-866-784-8937) or
1-800-LUNG-USA (1-800-586-4872)
Information on tobacco use and smoking cessation counseling by nurses, therapists, and smoking cessation counselors.

National Cancer Institute
http://www.cancer.gov
(use the search term "smoking")
Information and fact sheet on the harms of smoking and the benefits of quitting.

Nicotine Anonymous
http://www.nicotine-anonymous.org
A nonprofit twelve-step fellowship of men and women helping each other live nicotine-free lives.

SmokeEnders
http://www.smokenders.com
A self-study kit that includes seven weeks of seminars on audiotape, interactive workbook, and counseling services.

SmokeFree.gov
http://www.smokefree.gov
1-800-QUIT-NOW
A step-by-step guide to quitting offering a live chat option (online instant message) with a counselor and telephone counseling.

Way2Quit
http://www.way2quit.com
Information about the effects of tobacco and tips and steps to help with smoking cessation.

Stroke

American Stroke Association
http://www.strokeassociation.org
A division of the American Heart Association
that provides information and support to
stroke patients and their families.

American Stroke Foundation
http://www.americanstroke.org
Support for stroke survivors and their
caregivers.

Brain Attack Coalition
http://www.stroke-site.org
Resources from a coalition of professional
and government organizations dedicated to
providing quality treatment to patients.

The Internet Stroke Center
http://www.strokecenter.org
A directory of stroke centers offering a
life-after-stroke video series, caregiving,
resources to help children understand, and
extensive suggestions for home care.

**National Institute of Neurological Disorders
and Stroke**
http://www.ninds.nih.gov
Educational materials to improve stroke
awareness and provide information on
clinical trials.

National Stroke Association
http://www.stroke.org
Provides education and programs focused
on prevention, treatment, rehabilitation, and
support for all persons impacted by stroke.

PAD Coalition
http://www.stroke.org
Coordinated by the Vascular Disease
Foundation, the coalition is an alliance of
leading health organizations, vascular health
professional societies, and government
agencies united to raise public and health
professional awareness about lower
extremity peripheral arterial disease (PAD).

Vascular Disease Foundation
http://www.vdf.org
Nonprofit organization focused on vascular
diseases with the sole purpose of providing
public education and improving awareness
about vascular diseases.

Health Insurance

**Center for Consumer Information and
Insurance Oversight (CCIIIO)**
http://cciio.cms.gov
CCIIO is an arm of the U.S. Department of
Health and Human Services responsible
for implementing the Affordable Care Act.
This site provides consumer support and
information on its programs and initiatives,
such as working with state and local
governments to comply with new regulations
and protect consumers.

Foundation for Health Coverage Education
http://coverageforall.org
Assistance in finding affordable health
insurance coverage.

Healthcare and You Coalition
http://www.health careandyou.org
Formed by a group of consumer, patient, and
health care organizations to provide "easy
to understand" information about the health
care law and its impact on consumers.

Medicare.gov
http://www.medicare.gov
Updates, tools, and information about
Medicare.

National Association of Insurance Commissioners and The Center for Insurance Policy and Research
http://www.naic.org
Information about health care reform, options for finding affordable care with and without federal and state assistance, and links to each state's insurance commission for region-specific information.

Prescription Assistance

NeedyMeds.org
http://www.needymeds.org
A comprehensive database of free and low-cost prescription medicine programs as well as a prescription discount card, disease-based patient assistance resources, a database of state resources that help people apply for prescription assistance, and federal guidelines for determining Medicare and Medicaid eligibility.

Partnership for Prescription Assistance
http://www.pparx.org
Assists qualifying patients without prescription drug coverage to get for free or nearly free the medicines they need. The site also features a free and low-cost medical clinic finder, information about prescription savings cards, information about Medicare and Medicaid state child health insurance programs (CHIPs), and information about medication coupons.

RxAssist.org
http://rxassist.org
Offers resources for finding and applying for prescription assistance programs and provides a searchable database of programs offered by the states and pharmaceutical companies to help offset or eliminate the costs of medications for those who qualify. The site also provides help in understanding federal guidelines for Medicare and Medicaid and guidance in deciding which Medicare program is right for you. RxAssist.org also offers its own drug discount card for people who don't have prescription insurance.

Healthier Hearts for the Next Generation

Campaign for Tobacco-Free Kids
http://www.tobaccofreekids.org
A leading force in the fight to reduce tobacco use and its deadly toll in the United States and around the world.

Dr. Susan's Fit and Fun Family Action Plan
Dr. Bartell's easy and fun, step-by-step guide to help parents and grandparents to create a healthier home and more energetic kids.

Dr. Susan's Girls-Only Weight Loss Guide: The Easy, Fun Way to Look and Feel Good!
Written with the help of a dozen teenage girls, this book provides self-esteem affirming and body image building ways to lose weight healthily and without developing an eating disorder.

Let's Move
http://www.letsmove.gov
A comprehensive initiative launched by First Lady Michelle Obama, dedicated to solving the problem of obesity within a generation.

Mended Little Hearts

http://mendedlittlehearts.org

A support program for parents of children with heart defects and heart disease. Offering resources and a caring support network as families find answers and move forward to find healing and hope.

Spark Teens

http://www.sparkteens.com

An interactive website offering nutrition, health and fitness support, and tools to help teens lead healthier and happier lives.

WebMD Fit Kids

http://fit.webmd.com/kids

An interactive website for kids and teens designed to empower kids to take responsibility for their own health, including nutrition, exercise, mood, and sleep.

References

1. Canto JG, Shlipak MG, Rogers WJ, et al. Prevalence, clinical characteristics, and mortality among patients with myocardial infarction presenting without chest pain. JAMA 2000; 283: 3223–9.

2. Serruys PW, Unger F, Sousa JE, Jatene A, Bonnier HJ, Schönberger JP, Buller N, Bonser R, van den Brand MJ, van Herwerden LA, Morel MA, van Hout BA, Arterial Revascularization Therapies Study Group. Comparison of coronary-artery bypass surgery and stenting for the treatment of multivessel disease. N Engl J Med. 2001;344:1117–24.

3. Boden WE, O'Rourke RA, Teo KK, Hartigan PM, Maron DJ, Kostuk WJ, Knudtson M, Dada M, Casperson P, Harris CL, Chaitman BR, Shaw L, Gosselin G, Nawaz S, Title LM, Gau G, Blaustein AS, Booth DC, Bates ER, Spertus JA, Berman DS, Mancini GB, Weintraub WS. COURAGE Trial Research Group. Optimal medical therapy with or without PCI for stable coronary disease. N Engl J Med. 2007;356:1503–1516. (PG 19)

4. Pepine CJ, Abrams J, Marks RG, Morris JJ, Scheidt SS, Handberg E. Characteristics of a contemporary population with angina pectoris. TIDES Investigators. Am J Cardiol. 1994;74:226–31.

5. Knowler WC, Barrett-Connor E, Fowler SE, Hamman RF, Lachin JM, Walker EA, Nathan DM; Diabetes Prevention Program Research Group. Reduction in the incidence of Type 2 diabetes with lifestyle intervention or metformin. N Engl J Med. 2002;346:393–403.

6. Stuart RJ, Ellestad MH: National survey of exercise stress testing facilities. Chest 1980;77:94–7.

7. Randall C. Thompson, MD, and S. James Cullom, PhD. Issues regarding radiation dosage of cardiac nuclear and radiography procedures. J Nucl Cardiol 2006;13:19–23.

8. Frye RL, August P, Brooks MM, Hardison RM, Kelsey SF, MacGregor JM, Orchard TJ, Chaitman BR, Genuth SM, Goldberg SH, Hlatky MA, Jones TL, Molitch ME, Nesto RW, Sako EY, Sobel BE. A randomized trial of therapies for Type 2 diabetes and coronary artery disease, BARI 2D Study Group. N Engl J Med. 2009;360:2503–15. *Also see reference 3.*

9. G.J.W. Bech, B. De Bruyne, N.H.J. Pijls et al. Fractional flow reserve to determine the appropriateness of angioplasty in moderate coronary stenosis: a randomized trial. Circulation 2001;103:2928–34.

10. Tonino PA, De Bruyne B, Pijls NH, Siebert U, Ikeno F, van' t Veer M, Klauss V, Manoharan G, Engstrøm T, Oldroyd KG, Ver Lee PN, MacCarthy PA, Fearon WF; FAME Study Investigators. Fractional flow reserve versus angiography for guiding percutaneous coronary intervention. N Engl J Med. 2009 Jan 15;360(3):213–24.

11. Pijls NH, van Schaardenburgh P, Manoharan G, Boersma E, Bech JW, van't Veer M, Bär F, Hoorntje J, Koolen J, Wijns W, de Bruyne B. Percutaneous coronary intervention of functionally nonsignificant stenosis: 5-year follow-up of the DEFER Study. J Am Coll Cardiol. 2007 May 29;49(21):2105–11.

12. Jeremias A, Kutscher S, Haude M, Heinen D, Holtmann G, Senf W, Erbel R. Non-ischemic chest pain induced by coronary interventions: a prospective study comparing coronary angioplasty and stent implantation. Circulation. 1998;98:2656–8.

13. Wharton, TP. The Case for Community Hospital Angioplasty. Circulation. 2005;112:3509–34.

14. Khadour FH, Fu Y, Chang WC, Ma X, Mark D, Granger CB, Topol EJ, Califf RM, Armstrong PW, for the GUSTO IIb Investigators. Impact of on-site cardiac interventional facilities on management and outcomes of patients with acute coronary syndromes. Can J Cardiol. 2003; 19: 257–263.

15. Levine GN, Steinke EE, Bakaeen FG, Bozkurt B, Cheitlin MD, Conti JB, Foster E, Jaarsma T, Kloner RA, Lange RA, Lindau ST, Maron BJ, Moser DK, Ohman EM, Seftel AD, Stewart WJ; on behalf of the American Heart Association Council on Clinical Cardiology; Council on Cardiovascular Nursing; Council on Cardiovascular Surgery and Anesthesia, and Council on Quality of Care and Outcomes Research. Sexual activity and cardiovascular disease. A scientific statement from the American Heart Association. Circulation 2012;125:1058–72.

16. Heart Protection Study Collaborative Group. Effects on 11-year mortality and morbidity of lowering LDL cholesterol with simvastatin for about 5 years in 20 536 high-risk individuals: A randomised controlled trial. Lancet 2011;378:2013–20.

17. Ridker PM, Danielson E, Fonseca FA, Genest J, Gotto AM Jr, Kastelein JJ, Koenig W, Libby P, Lorenzatti AJ, MacFadyen JG, Nordestgaard BG, Shepherd J, Willerson JT, Glynn RJ. JUPITER Study Group. Rosuvastatin to prevent vascular events in men and women with elevated C-reactive protein. N Engl J Med. 2008;359:2195–207.

18. Leeper NJ, Ardehali R, deGoma EM, Heidenreich PA. Statin use in patients with extremely low low-density lipoprotein levels is associated with improved survival. Circulation 2007;116:613–8.

19. Lehman R, Krumholz HM. Tight control of blood glucose in long standing Type 2 diabetes. Brit Med J 2009;338:b1915.

20. Law M, Wald N, Morris J. Lowering blood pressure to prevent myocardial infarction and stroke: a new preventive strategy. Health Technol Assess 2003;7:1–94.

21. Chobanian AV, Bakris GL, Black HR, et al. Seventh report of the Joint National Committee on Prevention, Detection, Evaluation, and Treatment of High Blood Pressure. Hypertension 2003;42:1206–52.

22. Mostofsky E, Maclure M, Sherwood JB, Tofler GH, Muller JE, Mittleman MA. Risk of Acute Myocardial Infarction After the Death of a Significant Person in One's Life: The Determinants of Myocardial Infarction Onset Study. Circulation 2012;125:491–6.

23. Fiuzat M, Shaw LK, Thomas L, Felker GM, O'Connor CM. United States stock market performance and acute myocardial infarction rates in 2008–2009 (from the Duke Databank for Cardiovascular Disease). Am J Cardiol. 2010;106:1545–9.

24. Gautam S, Menachem J, Srivastav SK, Delafontaine P, Irimpen A. Effect of Hurricane Katrina on the incidence of acute coronary syndrome at a primary angioplasty center in New Orleans. Disaster Med Public Health Prep. 2009;3:144–50.

25. Nakagawa I, Nakamura K, Oyama M, Yamazaki O, Ishigami K, Tsuchiya Y, Yamamoto M. Long-term effects of the Niigata-Chuetsu earthquake in Japan on acute myocardial infarction mortality: an analysis of death certificate data. Heart. 2009;24:2009–13.

26. Pereg D, Gow R, Mosseri M, Lishner M, Ricder M, Van Uum S, Koren G. Hair cortisol and the risk for acute myocardial infarction in adult men. Stress. 2011;1:73–81.

27. Bodis J, Boncz I, Kriszbacher I. Permanent stress may be the trigger of an acute myocardial infarction on the first work-day of the week. Int J Cardiol. 2010;144:423–5.

28. Shen BJ, Avivi YE, Todaro JF, Spiro A 3rd, Laurenceau JP, Ward KD, Niaura R. Anxiety characteristics independently and prospectively predict myocardial infarction in men the unique contribution of anxiety among psychologic factors. J Am Coll Cardiol. 2008;51:113–9.

29. Haskell WL, Lee IM, Pate RR, Powell KE, Blair SN, Reginaldlin BA, Macera CA, Heath GW, Thompson PD, Bauman A; American College of Sports Medicine; American Heart Association. Physical activity and public health. Updated recommendation for adults from the American College of Sports Medicine and the American Heart Association. Circulation 2007;116:1081–93.

30. Kris-Etherton PM, Harris WS, Appel LJ; Nutrition Committee. Fish consumption, fish oil, omega-3 fatty acids, and cardiovascular disease. Circulation. 2002;106:2747–57.

31. 31. Knoops KT, de Groot LC, Kromhout D, et al. Mediterranean diet, lifestyle factors, and 10-year mortality in elderly European men and women: The HALE project. JAMA. 2004;292:1433–9.

32. Kris-Etherton PM, Lichtenstein AH, Howard BV, et al; Nutrition Committee of the American Heart Association Council on Nutrition, Physical Activity, and Metabolism. Antioxidant vitamin supplements and cardiovascular disease. Circulation. 2004;110:637–41.

33. Sacks FM, Svetkey LP, Vollmer WM, et al. DASH-Sodium Collaborative Research Group. Effects on blood pressure of reduced dietary sodium and the Dietary Approaches to Stop Hypertension (DASH) diet. N Engl J Med. 2001;344(1):3–10.

34. Mukamal KJ, Chen CM, Sowmya RR, Breslow RA. Alcohol consumption and cardiovascular mortality among U.S. adults, 1987 to 2002 J Am Coll Cardiol 2010;55:1328–35.

35. Klatsky AL, Friedman GD, Armstrong MA, Kipp H. Wine, liquor, beer, and mortality. Am J Epidemiol 2003;158:585–95.

36. Corrao G, Bagnardi V, Zambon A, La Vecchia C. A meta-analysis of alcohol consumption and the risk of 15 diseases. Prev Med 2004;38:613–9.

37. Chen WY, Rosner B, Hankinson SE, Colditz GA, Willett WC. Moderate alcohol consumption during adult life, drinking patterns, and breast cancer risk. JAMA. 2011;306:1884–90.

38. Hajek P, Taylor T, McRobbie H. The effect of stopping smoking on perceived stress levels. Addiction. 2010;105:1466–71.

39. Thom T, Haase N, Rosamond W, Howard VJ, Rumsfeld J, Manolio T, Zheng ZJ, Flegal K, O'Donnell C, Kittner S, Lloyd-Jones D, Goff DC Jr, Hong Y, Adams R, Friday G, Furie K, Gorelick P, Kissela B, Marler J, Meigs J, Roger V, Sidney S, Sorlie P, Steinberger J, Wasserthiel-Smoller S, Wilson M, Wolf P; American Heart Association Statistics Committee and Stroke Statistics Subcommittee. Heart disease and stroke statistics—2006 update: a report from the American Heart Association Statistics Committee and Stroke Statistics Subcommittee. Circulation. 2006;113:e85–151.

40. Taira DA, Seto TB, Ho KK, Krumholz HM, Cutlip DE, Berezin R, Kuntz RE, Cohen DJ. Impact of smoking on health-related quality of life after percutaneous coronary revascularization. Circulation 2000;102:1369–74.)

Index

—— A ——

ABC plan for diabetics, 164
abdominal aortic aneurysms, 211–212
ACE (angiotensin-converting enzyme)
    inhibitors, 168, 169
acid reflux, 8–9
Adenosine, 40
AHA (American Heart Association),
    182
AHRQ (U.S. Agency for Healthcare
    Research and Quality) Clinical
    Practice Guideline on Smoking
    Cessation, 217
alcohol intake
    amount you can drink, 207
    antithrombotic effects of, 208
    benefits of moderate, 208–209
    breast cancer and, 210–211
    French paradox, 209–210
    high blood pressure and, 167
    moderate, 208
    risk factors of, 206
    your comfort level with, 206–207
    your experience with, 206–209
allergies, 122–123, 128
alpha-agonists, 169
alpha-blockers, 169
American Heart Association (AHA),
    182
angiograms. See coronary angiograms
angioplasty (percutaneous coronary
    intervention)
    alternatives to, 164–165
    clot extraction during, 128
    discomfort during, 109
    emergency, 126
    following coronary angiograms,
        71–72

healing after, 118–119
how they work, 101–105
pain during, 110
risks/complications of, 113–115,
    120–125
stents for, 53–54
unavailability of, 128–129
what to expect during, 107–109
when to have, 96
angiotensin II-receptor blockers
    (ARBs), 168, 169
angiotensin-converting enzyme (ACE)
    inhibitors, 168, 169
anti-cholesterol agents, 151
anti-platelet agents, 150–151
anxiety, anticipatory, 175
aorta, 122, 211–212
aortic valve, 45
ARBs (angiotensin II-receptor
    blockers), 168, 169
arrhythmias, 213
arterial occlusion/blockage. See
    blockages (arterial)
arteries, hardening/narrowing of,
    11–12, 213
artificial respiration, 226. See also
    cardiopulmonary resuscitation
    (CPR)
aspirin, 66, 115, 118–119, 127–128,
    150
atherosclerosis, 213

—— B ——

balloon angioplasty. See angioplasty
    (percutaneous coronary
    intervention)
beta blockers, 168, 169, 179
bleeding, 84, 121–122, 151

blockages (arterial). *See also* coronary
  artery disease (CAD)
  benefits of fast removal, 127
  categories of, 94–95
  causes of, 9–10
  critical versus noncritical, 36
  degree of blockage and symptom,
    10
  detection during stress tests, 35, 41
  hemodynamic significance of, 95
  locating, 87
  in main arteries, 8–9
  partial, 15–16
  preventing worsening/new, 63
  risk factors for, 50
  treating multiple, 105–106
  treatment options, 87–89
  when to fix, 96
blockages (of heart valves), 45
blood clots (thrombosis), 9–10, 12,
    118–119, 127–128. *See also*
    blockages (arterial)
blood pressure, high. *See* high blood
    pressure (HBP)
blood sugar, 160, 195
blood thinners. *See* medications
blood transfusions, 122
blood vessel damage, 123, 212–213
BMI (body mass index), 200
body mass index (BMI), 200
broken-heart syndrome (Takotsubo
    cardiomyopathy), 179
bypass surgery
  benefits of, 89–90, 91, 145
  blockage development in bypasses,
    135–136
  description, 131–133
  emergency, 129
  indications for, 99, 124, 130–131,
    148
  memory loss after, 134–135
  minimally invasive, 135
  multiple bypasses, 135
  quitting smoking and, 215
  recovery from, 133–134
  returning to exercise after, 136–137
  returning to work after, 138
  as risk factor, 22, 65
  veins used for, 133
  without symptoms, 161

—— C ——

calcifications of coronary arteries, 46,
    48
calcium channel blockers, 169
cancer, 210–211, 219
cardiac cocktail, 148, 149–152. *See also*
    medications
cardiac rehabilitation, 144–145
cardiologists, 28–32, 51–52
cardiopulmonary resuscitation (CPR),
    6, 223–226
cardiovascular disease, 208
CAT scans, 46, 48, 52–53
cholesterol levels, 11, 23, 25, 151,
    153–156, 164
  HDL and LDL, 25–26, 151, 156–
    157, 194, 200, 208, 213
Clinical Practice Guideline on
    Smoking Cessation, 217
clot busters, 128
clots, 9–10, 12, 118–119. *See also*
    blockages (arterial)
cold laser therapy, 218
conscious sedation, 78
contrast dye, 48, 122–125
coronaries. *See* heart attacks
coronary angiograms, 48
  access sites, 79–80, 83–84, 85, 86
  anxiety before, 80
  complications and precautions after,
    82–86
  complications of, 82–86
  description of procedure, 68–72
  effectiveness of, 98
  emergency, 100
  following abnormal stress test,
    49–50
  hospital stays after, 81
  medications administered during,
    80
  reasons for, 64–65
  recovery from, 86
  risks of, 51
  tube and catheter placement, 69,
    73–74
  tube placement, 72–73
  what to expect, 75–79
coronary angioplasty. *See* angioplasty
    (percutaneous coronary
    intervention)

coronary artery disease (CAD). *See also* blockages (arterial)
  benefits of quitting smoking, 217
  calcifications, 46
  causes of, 21–22
  curing versus controlling, 62–63
  description, 18
  with hypertension, 169
  medications for, 65–66
  risk factors, 22–26, 152, 163, 174, 200, 207, 212
  sexual activity with, 138–139
  stress tests for (*See* stress tests)
cortisol level, 175
CPR. *See* cardiopulmonary resuscitation (CPR)
C-reactive protein (CRP), 151

—— D ——

dairy products, 192
DASH diet, 198–199
defibrillation, 224, 226. *See also* cardiopulmonary resuscitation (CPR)
depression, 139
DHA (docosahexaenoic acid), 197
diabetes
  ABC plan, 164
  controlling, 161
  deaths related to, 159
  description, 159–160
  effects on heart of, 160–161
  fish, 197
  hemoglobin testing and, 164
  medications for controlling, 152
  related medical issues, 163
  resources, 231
  as risk factor for coronary artery disease, 11, 23, 25, 158–164
  risk factors, 24, 158–164, 163
  risk factors for, 24, 163
  silent heart attacks and, 7
  testing glucose blood level, 162–163
  Type 1 and 2, 160
diastolic blood pressure, 168
diet/nutrition. *See also* overweight/obesity; weight loss
  after coronary angiogram/angioplasties, 85
  calories, 202–204

changing to healthy, 189–196
cholesterol-containing foods, 194–195
DASH diet, 198–199
fats, 192, 205
fiber, 193, 201
fish oil supplements, 197
foods to limit/avoid, 193–195
fruit, 192, 204
glycemic index (GI), 198
high-cholesterol foods, 154
portion control, 196
processed foods, 193
protein, 192–193, 196, 205
resources, 229–230
salt, 64, 167, 193
sugar, 195
vegetables, 192, 196, 204
vitamin and mineral supplements, 198
whole grain foods, 192, 196
differential uptake, 41
direct renin inhibitors, 169
diuretics, 168
Dobutamine, 41
docosahexaenoic acid (DHA), 197
doctor review websites, 31–32
drug interactions, 149–150
drug-eluting stents, 114, 117–119
dual anti-platelet therapy, 150–151

—— E ——

ECG. *See* electrocardiography (ECG or EKG)
echocardiograms, 37, 44, 47
EF (ejection fraction), 44–45, 47
eicosapentaenoic acid (EPA), 197
ejection fraction (EF), 44–45, 47
electrocardiography (ECG or EKG), 34, 36–37, 43, 46–47
emergency situations/procedures
  after stent placement, 115
  angiograms as, 81, 100
  angioplasty as, 42, 100, 126–129
  avoiding, 179
  bypass surgery, 124
  instructions for CPR in, 223–226
  reactions to medications, 118
  retroperitoneal bleed, 121
  waiting too long to see a doctor, 126–127

when to call 911, 6, 86, 90, 118, 224, 225
when to see your doctor, 16–17, 18, 19, 83–84
Environmental Protection Agency (EPA), 197
EPA (eicosapentaenoic acid), 197
EPA (Environmental Protection Agency), 197
exercise. *See also* rehabilitation after heart attacks
    aerobic, 183
    after stent placement, 136–137
    age and fitness/strength, 188–189
    benefits of, 181
    as cause of chest discomfort, 17
    chest pain/pressure during/after, 13–16, 32–33
    determination of fitness for, 38
    how to get started, 181–182, 183–184
    improving balance, 188
    joining a gym, 187
    lack of, 12
    length of sessions, 184–185
    physical activity, 230
    professional trainers, 188
    recommendations after heart attack for, 180–181
    reducing high blood pressure with, 166–167
    resources, 230
    returning to, 136–137
    staying motivated, 185–187
    strength training, 183, 185
    stress tests with (*See* stress tests)
    stretching, 183
    walking, 183–184
    for weight loss, 201
exertion, non-exercise types of, 17

—— F ——

family issues, 55–60, 130
FDA (Food and Drug Administration), 197
FFR (fractional flow reserve) test, 96, 98–99
fitness, 38
fractional flow reserve (FFR) test, 96, 98–99

—— G ——

genetics, 22, 24
Global Utilization of Strategies to Open Occluded Arteries (GUSTO) IIb, 129
glucose (sugar), 160, 162–163, 164. *See also* diabetes
glycemic index (GI), 198

—— H ——

hard plaque, 48
hardening of the arteries, 11–12, 48
HBP. *See* high blood pressure (HBP)
HDL and LDL cholesterol, 151, 156–157, 194, 200, 208, 213
health insurance, 232–233
health resources, 227
heart
    alcohol intake and healthy, 207
    complications of coronary angiograms for, 82
    diabetes effects on, 160–161
    high blood pressure effects on, 166
    potential damage to, 8–9
    resources for healthier, 227–229, 233–244
    smoking effects on, 212
heart attacks
    activity after, 180–188 (*See also* exercise)
    during angioplasty, 122
    damage to heart from, 42
    recovery from, 139
    rehabilitation after, 144–145
    restarting the heart, 226 (*See also* cardiopulmonary resuscitation (CPR); defibrillation)
    risk of sexual activity for, 138–139
    signs/symptoms, 4–5
    during sports events, 178–179
    stress-related, 173, 175
    triggers and warning signs of, 18
    warning signs, 16–17
    what to do, 6
    without symptoms, 5–6, 7
heart catheterization (coronary angiogram). *See* coronary angiograms
heart disease risk factors, 10–11, 25, 138–139, 212–213

heart valve blockages, 45
heart-lung machines, 132–133
Heart♥SMART program, 143, 189–196,
    206–209
hemodynamic flow/significance, 95,
    98–99. *See also* fractional flow
    reserve (FFR) test
herbal therapy for smoking cessation,
    218–219
high blood pressure (HBP)
    coronary artery disease and high, 23
    DASH diet for, 198–199
    with diabetes, 164
    effects on body of, 166
    managing, without medications, 165
    medications for, 152, 168–169
    reasons for medications with
        normal, 169
    risk factors for, 163
    salt intake and, 64
    understanding the numbers, 168
    ways of reducing, 166–167
    ways to reduce, 26
high-density lipoprotein cholesterol.
    See HDL and LDL cholesterol
hormonal changes, 175
hydrogenated oils, 194
hypertension. *See* high blood pressure
    (HBP)
hypnosis for smoking cessation, 218

——— I ———

infections, 85, 226
in-stent restenosis, 113–114
insulin, 160, 195
insurance coverage, 54
internal mammary artery bypass
    surgery, 132
intravascular ultrasound (IVUS), 100
invasive (interventional) cardiologists,
    51–52
invasive procedures, 68
IVUS (intravascular ultrasound), 100

——— J ———

journaling, 145–146

——— K ———

kidney damage, 22, 122–123, 124–125,
    155

kidney function assessment, 53

——— L ———

LDL (low-density lipoprotein)
    cholesterol. *See* HDL and LDL
    cholesterol
leg pain, 22
lifestyle issues, 12, 23–24, 26, 64, 97,
    144, 179. *See also Heart♥*SMART
    program; weight loss
liver damage, 155

——— M ———

maximal work capacity (peak
    functional capacity), 38
meals/snacks, 191–192
medication-coated stents, 114,
    117–119
medications
    aspirin, 66, 115, 118–119, 127–128,
        150
    for blood pressure therapy, 66
    blood thinners, 66, 115, 118, 150
    Brilinta (ticagrelor), 115, 118,
        150–151
    cardiac cocktail, 148, 149–152
    Chantix (varenicline), 217
    Crestor (rosuvastatin), 151
    for diabetes control, 161
    drug interactions, 149–150
    effectiveness of, 90–91
    Effient (prasugrel), 115, 118,
        150–151
    feeling effects of, 155–156
    for high blood pressure (HBP), 167,
        168–169
    Lescol (fluvastatin), 151
    Lipitor (atorvastatin), 151, 153
    Livalo (pitavastatin), 151
    Mevacor (lovastation), 151
    Mucomyst (N-acetylcysteine), 125
    optimal medical therapy, 97
    for pain, 78
    as part of treatment, 63–64
    Plavix (clopidogrel), 66, 115, 118,
        150–151
    Pravachol (pravastatin), 151
    side effects of, 148–149, 154–155
    for smoking cessation, 217–218
    statins (*See* statins)

for stress tests, 40
Zocor (simvastatin), 151
Zyban (bupropion), 217
metabolic disorders, 159
minorities health resources, 229
mitral valve, 45
mouth-to-mouth breathing, 226
muscle weakness, 155
myoglobin, 155

—— N ——

nuclear imaging material, 37, 40–41
nutrition therapy, 195. *See also* diet/
nutrition

—— O ——

occlusions, arterial. *See* blockages
(arterial)
omega-3 fatty acids, 197
optimal (target) heart rate, 34, 40
optimal medical therapy, 97, 169
osteoporosis, 184
overweight/obesity, 11, 25, 64, 163. *See
also* diet/nutrition; weight loss
oxygen concentration, 213

—— P ——

PAD (peripheral artery disease), 22,
23, 24, 159
pain
after coronary angiograms, 82,
83–84
chest pain/pressure during/after
exercise, 15
during coronary angiograms, 78
leg, 22
stretch pain after stent procedure,
110–111
tolerance for, 7
pancreas, 160
partially hydrogenated oils, 194
PCI. *See* angioplasty (percutaneous
coronary intervention)
peak functional capacity (maximal
work capacity), 38
percutaneous coronary intervention.
See angioplasty (percutaneous
coronary intervention)
peripheral artery disease (PAD), 22,
23, 24, 159

peripheral vascular disease (PVD),
212
Persantine, 40
plaque, 9–10
in aorta, 122
cracking of, 103–104, 104–105
effects of buildup of, 11–12
hard/soft, 48
inflammation from, 11–12
ruptures of, 11–12
snowplow effect, 123–124
stopping accumulation of, 63
platelet clumping, 213
pleiotropic effects of statins, 157–158
prescription assistance, 233
preventive medicine, 195
PVD (peripheral vascular disease),
212

—— R ——

radiation exposure, 37, 48
Regadenoson, 40
rehabilitation after heart attacks, 133,
144–145. *See also* exercise
resveratrol, 210
retroperitoneal bleed, 121–122
rhabdomyolysis, 155
Rotablator, 105

—— S ——

saphenous vein bypass surgery, 132
saturated fats, 194
sedation, 78, 107
sexual activity, 12, 138–139
side effects of medications, 148–149,
154–155, 156
silent heart attacks, 7
smoking
effects of, 211–215
high blood pressure and, 167
nicotine, 213–215
nicotine effects, 213–215
as risk factor for coronary artery
disease, 22, 24–25
before stress tests, 34
smoking cessation, 64, 215–220, 231.
See also smoking
acupuncture for, 218
electronic cigarettes, 219
natural methods for, 218–219

Nicotine Anonymous (NicA), 216
nicotine replacement therapy, 216, 217
prescription drugs for, 217–218
programs for, 215–216
reasons for, 212–214
resources, 231
success rates, 220
weight gain with, 220
snacks/meals, 191–192
snowplow effect (plaque), 123–124
soft plaque, 48
sonograms. *See* ultrasound
statins, 65, 151
benefits of, 153–154
how they work, 157–158
with normal cholesterol level, 153–156
side effects of, 154–155, 156
stent thrombosis
risk factors, 118–119
stents, 65
alternatives to, 164–165
benefits of, 125–126
blood thinners after insertion of, 53–54
description, 111–112, 115–116
drug-eluting, 114, 117–119
effectiveness of, 89–90
permanence of, 113
placement of, 103–104
re-blockage of (restenosis), 161
recovery time, 136–137
snowplow effect, 123–124
stress reduction
resources, 231
stress reduction techniques, 55–56, 58, 176, 177–178, 231
stress tests
accuracy of, 35–36, 95, 96
chest discomfort during, 41
description, 33–35
false negatives and positives, 36–37
with fractional flow reserve test, 98–99
medications used during, 40–41
optimal (target) heart rate, 34, 40
pharmacologic, 39, 40–41
physical limitations for performing, 38–39

recommendations for abnormal results, 49
smoking/eating/caffeine intake before, 34
understanding results, 50
stress/stressors
acute/chronic, 173
blood pressure elevation with, 16–19
broken-heart syndrome (Takotsubo cardiomyopathy), 179
how to recognize, 172–174
mechanism of triggering heart attacks, 174–175
physiological responses to, 179
relationships, 58–59
signs/symptoms of experiencing, 174
smoking as, 214
stress-related heart attacks, 175
stretch pain after stent procedure, 110–111
stroke information, 232
strokes, 232
during angioplasty, 122
risk factors, 25, 26, 166
statins for, 65, 153
sugar (blood level of). *See* diabetes; glucose (sugar)
support network
family and friends, 55–60
problems of, 59–60
professional, 58–59
symptoms
determining treatment options by, 88
erratic, 16
experienced by men, 7
experienced by women and men, 7
heart valve blockages, 45
identifying triggers of, 50
nicotine withdrawal, 214
typical appearance of, 45
systolic blood pressure, 165, 168

—— T ——

Takotsubo cardiomyopathy (broken-heart syndrome), 179
target (optimal) heart rate, 34, 40
thrombosis, stent, 114–115,

118–119, 179. *See also* blood clots
  (thrombosis)
treatment
  angioplasty (percutaneous coronary
    intervention) (*See* angioplasty
    (percutaneous coronary
    intervention))
  bypass surgery (*See* bypass surgery)
  deciding on, 100
  dissolving blood clots, 127–128
  effectiveness of different, 90–91
  effects of delaying, 11
  optimal medical therapy, 97
  risk factors of options, 88
triglycerides, 163
two-person CPR, 225

—— U ——

ultrasound, 37, 41, 43–44, 47, 100
U.S. Agency for Healthcare Research
  and Quality (AHRQ) Clinical
  Practice Guideline on Smoking
  Cessation, 217

—— V ——

vegetarian proteins, 192–193
vomiting, 226

—— W ——

warning signs of heart attacks, 19. *See
  also* emergency situations
weight loss. *See also* diet/nutrition;
  overweight/obesity
  after quitting smoking, 220
  body mass index (BMI), 200
  calorie consumption, 202–204
  calories in drinks, 200–201
  determining need for, 199
  exercise, 201
  increasing fiber intake, 201
  professional support for, 202
  reducing high blood pressure with,
    166–167
  setting a goal, 201
  skipping meals, 201
  tips for, 204–205
women
  health resources for, 229
women's health, 229

—— X ——

X-rays, 71

About the Authors and Contributors

Authors

Allen Jeremias, MD, MSc, is an Associate Professor of Medicine and a practicing interventional cardiologist at Stony Brook University Medical School in Stony Brook, New York. He is the Medical Director of the Cardiac Intensive Care and the Cardiac Acute Care units at Stony Brook University Medical Center. He is an internationally recognized researcher with numerous publications in the area of interventional cardiology and the editor of *Cardiac Intensive Care,* the only major textbook on that topic. Over the past four years, he has been recognized by Castle Connolly as a Top Doctor in the New York Metro Area.

Susan Bartell, PsyD, is a nationally recognized psychologist, speaker, and award-winning author of seven books. She has been helping people take control of their physical and emotional health for over twenty years. She specializes in educating people about healthy lifestyle, life balance, and stress reduction. She has a private practice in the New York tristate area, counseling people of all ages in areas related to health, weight loss, life balance, stress, anxiety, and depression. Dr. Bartell also lectures widely to varied groups, including corporate clients, on topics related to physical and emotional health. She is a recognized media expert and has been an expert contributor on many national television shows, including *The Today Show, The Early Show,* and *Good Morning America.* She is also a regular contributor to national media outlets including NBC, ABC, CBS, CNN, *USA Today,* and the *New York Times.*

Contributors

Teri Reilly, RD, CDN, CDE, is a registered dietitian, a medical nutrition therapist, and a certified diabetes educator who has worked in the field for more than twenty-five years. She works in the New York area as the Nutritionist and Diabetes Educator at Cardiovascular Medical Associates PC, an affiliate of Winthrop Heart and Vascular Institute University Hospital. Teri specializes in cardiovascular disease, diabetes, and weight management. She is a Certified Insulin Pump Trainer, and for almost ten years she has been a preceptor for student interns in the Long Island University Post Dietetic Intern Program. She holds a certificate of training in Adult Weight Management, awarded by the American Dietetic Association Commission on Dietetic Registration. Teri regularly provides presentations on a wide range of topics related to diet and nutrition.

Steve Panzik, MSPT, CSCS, is a licensed physical therapist and owner of Power Ten Fitness Club in Port Washington, New York. As an exercise physiologist he has worked in- and outpatient care with cardiac rehab at Temple University and Memorial Regional Hospital. Steve's degrees include a BS in exercise physiology and an MS in physical therapy. He was a Division I athlete, achieving four national championships and two Big East titles in rowing, and he was a member of the 1993 National Rowing Team. He is the men's and women's crew coach at Port Rowing on Long Island. Steve holds certifications in Pilates, golf-specific rehabilitation and fitness, as is a certified strength conditioning specialist. He has worked closely with Rich Dalatri of the New Jersey Nets to develop the Pilates for Athletes workouts and multiple speed and agility programs. Steve has led fitness segments on *The Today Show, Good Day New York,* and *The CW11 Morning News* and has been featured in *Newsday's Parent and Child* magazine and *Men's Journal.*